1,001 Days

Also by Sue Gerhardt

Why Love Matters
The Selfish Society

1,001 Days

How Our First Years Shape Our Lifelong Health

SUE GERHARDT

Cornerstone Press

CORNERSTONE PRESS

UK | USA | Canada | Ireland | Australia
India | New Zealand | South Africa

Cornerstone Press is part of the Penguin Random House group of companies whose addresses can be found at global.penguinrandomhouse.com

Penguin Random House UK,
One Embassy Gardens, 8 Viaduct Gardens, London SW11 7BW

penguin.co.uk

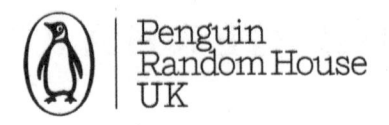

Penguin
Random House
UK

First published 2025
001

Copyright © Sue Gerhardt, 2025

The moral right of the author has been asserted

The image and text acknowledgements and permissions on pp. 263–4 constitute an extension of this copyright page

Penguin Random House values and supports copyright. Copyright fuels creativity, encourages diverse voices, promotes freedom of expression and supports a vibrant culture. Thank you for purchasing an authorised edition of this book and for respecting intellectual property laws by not reproducing, scanning or distributing any part of it by any means without permission. You are supporting authors and enabling Penguin Random House to continue to publish books for everyone. No part of this book may be used or reproduced in any manner for the purpose of training artificial intelligence technologies or systems. In accordance with Article 4(3) of the DSM Directive 2019/790, Penguin Random House expressly reserves this work from the text and data mining exception.

Set in 12/15.25pt Dante MT Std
Typeset by Jouve (UK), Milton Keynes
Printed and bound in Great Britain by Clays Ltd, Elcograf S.p.A.

The authorised representative in the EEA is Penguin Random House Ireland, Morrison Chambers, 32 Nassau Street, Dublin D02 YH68

A CIP catalogue record for this book is available from the British Library

ISBN 978–1–529–92867–9 (hardback)
ISBN 978–1–529–92868–6 (trade paperback)

Penguin Random House is committed to a sustainable future for our business, our readers and our planet. This book is made from Forest Stewardship Council® certified paper.

MIX
Paper | Supporting
responsible forestry
FSC® C018179

For my grandson, Luca

Everything should be as simple as possible, but not simpler.

(attributed to Albert Einstein)

Contents

Introduction: How to grow healthy humans — 1

PART ONE
Health Stories

1. Germs and genes — 11
2. Growing a person: a social, interactive view of health — 33

PART TWO
The Body Under Construction

3. Starting with cells — 61
4. Growing inside mother's body — 73
5. The post-natal cocoon — 101

PART THREE
When Things Go Wrong

6. Unprotected: stressful relationships and how they affect health — 139
7. Child poverty and health — 167

Conclusion

8. Future-proofing human beings — 195

Notes — 217
Epigraph and image credits — 263
Acknowledgements — 265
Index — 267

Introduction:

How to grow heathy humans

Babyhood and old age are seen as polar opposites and are rarely mentioned in the same breath. Yet they are profoundly linked. The earliest experiences we have as fetus and infant have lasting effects on our lives, particularly on our mental and physical health as adults.

I first came to understand these links in the 1990s and wrote about them in *Why Love Matters: How Affection Shapes a Baby's Brain*.[1] As I embarked on this new book, decades later, I wanted to focus less on the brain and mental health and more on physical health, once again exploring how very early events can shape health – especially our health after middle age.

What I didn't realise then was what a personal story this would turn out to be. As I started researching and talking to people about it, the first of my circle of friends and family developed a serious illness: my younger sister, Vicky, was diagnosed with a form of lymphoma or blood cancer, which was successfully treated. Then there was Harriet.

Harriet was a lynchpin of our friendly neighbourhood. Attractive, self-deprecating, warm and hospitable, we sometimes gathered at her house for a drink on bonfire night. There she would be, smoking her tiny roll-up cigarettes and making wry comments about the state of the world, or tactfully enquiring about other people's lives. She looked fit, slim and contented with her own life, so it was a shock to hear that she had developed lung cancer while only in her sixties.

One weekend, some of the residents of our street met up for an impromptu summer picnic on the scrubby common near our homes. An unexpected shower had made it so damp that we had to lay coats on the ground. As we passed around the crisps and home-made dips, I explained the theme of this book to her: that many adult illnesses were thought to be linked to early life experiences, often due to the mother's stress during pregnancy or postnatally affecting the baby's immune system. Immediately, Harriet responded: 'That's me.' She instantly recognised the possibility that her own difficult childhood may have played a part in her illness, just as much as lifestyle factors had, like smoking.

That was also the summer when it began to dawn on me that my generation of 'baby boomers' were starting to come face-to-face with the reality of ageing. There was more to come: first there were the unexpected deaths of iconic figures, such as the musician David Bowie, the actor Alan Rickman and the comedian Victoria Wood, all in their sixties. Then – closer to home – the toll mounted as other neighbours and friends died of things like pancreatic cancer, myeloma and heart disease, among them my close friend Dave, who had suffered from chronic obstructive pulmonary disease (COPD) and kidney failure for several years.

Around this time my own health started to fray at the edges too. Although I was researching and reading hundreds of scientific papers, it took me a while to realise that something had happened to my eyesight: a blood clot in one eye that was affecting my vision. Then I had another shock when, a year or two later, I was diagnosed with Parkinson's disease. I began to realise that I, too, had entered that stage of life where the body starts to fail.

But this book is not about the gloomy trials of old age.

Instead, it has a positive message. It suggests that, with a better understanding of the early roots of health and illness, we could target our efforts differently – both as adults seeking to safeguard our own health and as a society looking to create more effective ways to prevent chronic illness. It also suggests that things could be very different for future generations. As we begin to understand the links between early experience and later disease, the possibility of prevention becomes more compelling. It opens up new and exciting opportunities to reduce the number of people who develop cardiovascular disease, obesity, type-2 diabetes, depression and dementia – our number-one health problems, over and above the newly relevant challenge of pandemic viruses.

A clear but complex picture is emerging; there is no simple cause and effect that explains an individual's health outcomes. Every person's story is unique. For example, many factors came together to set my friend Dave up for ill health. His parents had little money (his father was a motor mechanic and his mother a cleaner); he described them as harsh parents with sharp tongues who often left him feeling humiliated and unloved, which, he regretfully worried, had an ongoing effect on his adult relationships. Their family food was cheap and filling. It did not feature any vegetables other than the potato. As Dave used to enjoy telling people, in an exaggerated Mancunian accent: 'My first meal was a chip.' And although he became a good cook in later life, Dave never gave up his taste for those familiar pies and chips.

People with a less auspicious start in life may not acquire the 'brain reserve' generated by positive early life experiences. Those who are held and touched, well fed, warm and emotionally secure are likely to have brains with more neuronal connections, less inflammation and a more robust immune system, which in turn delays the onset of the diseases of ageing. For people like Dave or Harriet, who also experienced stress in early life, or those who lost a parent in childhood, there may be less brain reserve and less resilience in the face of stress or infection.

Does that mean it is too late for those of us who recognise this may have been our own story? On the contrary, it gives us, as adults, more chance of using an awareness of our own particular vulnerability to illness to protect ourselves from the kinds of stress that can trigger it, just as we might use our knowledge of a family history of heart disease to guide us to regularly check our blood pressure. Knowing the history of your own first 1,001 days could motivate you more strongly to try to reduce the stress in your life – for example, by seeking help with stressful personal relationships, practising self-soothing techniques, or by collaborating with others to correct social injustices. Equally, it could lead to a greater willingness to take part in screening programmes, to reduce inflammation through your food choices, or just to act more promptly when symptoms appear.

If we could also find a way to pay more attention to these processes at the start of life – by promoting maternal well-being in pregnancy, supporting breastfeeding, and strengthening the early attachment relationships – we would not only help people to enjoy their lives but would also build positive 'health capital'. The possibility then opens up of reducing the number of people who get cardiovascular disease, obesity, depression, type 2 diabetes and other conditions.

The better we can understand the way these different factors affect us in the present, the more likely it is that we will be able to effectively prevent ill health. But this is a different way of approaching illness from the prevailing medical model, which focuses more narrowly on symptoms, diseases and cures. This book will argue that it is time to expand our thinking. We need to take on board the combined impact of the revolutionary changes that have been happening in a range of sciences, such as neuroscience, developmental psychology, microbiology and epigenetics, which point us to the importance of early experience in being resilient and healthy throughout our life. The knowledge these disciplines have been accumulating in recent decades is, however, mostly found in academic journals and is rarely made accessible to the casual reader. The intention of this book is to make their discoveries as clear as possible, without unnecessary jargon, so that we can see their implications more clearly.

Our current health systems do not, as yet, fully embrace the potential of prevention, especially the power to prevent future illness at the earliest stages of development. Although there are a few significant forms of early prevention, such as early programmes of vaccination in infancy and childhood and the monitoring of pregnant women's health, the idea of prevention is largely focused on stopping established unhealthy adult behaviours, such as smoking and weight gain.

This book explores some of the deep-rooted political and cultural issues that hinder us from acting on what developmental science is telling us. Some of these wider issues are about the stories by which we live our lives. For example, we take an individualistic framework for granted. Ill health tends to be seen as a result of the wrong 'lifestyle' choices, or as an individual struggle against adversity (as can be seen from headlines such as: 'Olivia Newton-John battling breast cancer again'). We hold fast to the idea that we can determine our lives through our own actions and free will – in fact, many believe this is 'the essence of humanness'.[2]

The possibility that our health and well-being depend on other people, particularly on events that occur in the earliest months of our lives, does not fit comfortably with Western thinking. Currently, few people recognise any link between their adult health concerns and what happened to them in the womb or as a baby. This book argues that this is a significant and neglected part of the picture. Each of us is made or grown by and with other people: we can never have unfettered freedom, nor can we single-handedly make ourselves who we are. As René Dubos, the Frenchman who pioneered ecological thinking, put it: 'each one of us is born with the potentiality to become several different persons but what we become depends on the conditions under which we develop'.[3]

This is turning out to be true of our health as well as our psychological selves. Each body develops in response to its environment. For example, it is well known that the individual's acquired immune system is 'a product of the types, strengths and number of infections, diseases and injuries encountered through life'.[4] What is less well known is that several other systems that play a part in regulating the body – such as our stress response, the vagal system, the gut microbiome and various neurotransmitter and hormone systems that we will cover in this book – can also develop differently in response to different experiences and environments, particularly in response to the nutritional and emotional care we receive early on in life.

This relatively new information suggests the need to update our established ways of thinking about health and illness. Predominant ideas of medicine are focused on eradicating germs, on new technical and surgical fixes, and on finding the genes involved in particular illnesses. These are all worthy goals, for which I am grateful, particularly as someone living with Parkinson's disease. It also makes sense for adults to adopt a healthy diet and exercise regime, and to stop smoking, to reduce our risk of falling ill. More than that, however, with a greater understanding of our individual health stories, we can be alert to the risks we face and become better able to make informed decisions about our health. But healthy aging also depends on health in infancy and childhood, factors that receive less attention.

Happily, more and more people in the medical profession are raising these issues – people like Richard Horton, 'activist' editor of the respected medical journal *The Lancet*, who has campaigned about the importance of nutrition, the need to reform our food system and to prioritise maternal and child healthcare; or the Cambridge University paediatrician Professor David Rowitch, who recently argued for a 'healthcare paradigm shift' towards preventive medicine, identifying the origins of disease early on in order to build health resilience. As he put it, somewhat pessimistically, 'Beginning disease prevention in middle age is not just closing the stable door after the horse has bolted; those horses have left the field and they're not coming back'.[5] These voices are getting louder.

As this book will make clear, it is way past time to listen to such voices. The growing pressures of climate overheating, unstable democracies, new pandemics and increasing social inequality are making it both more difficult yet more imperative to move away from short-sighted reactive behaviours and move towards long-term

Introduction

planning and thinking, if we are to create a healthy, resilient new generation. There is an urgent need to 'take control' of our global economy and of the environment if we are to have a viable future, but, equally, we need to ensure that new people who are born in the years to come are built for healthy lives.

Additionally, armed with new and consolidating information about the physiological systems that underpin and maintain health, we can all benefit by embracing a wider concept of medicine and a growing understanding of how to repair and restore some of our systems that may have developed poorly in early life.

The exciting thing is that we understand more than ever how this can be done.

PART ONE

Health Stories

1.

Germs and genes

'Such a tendency to see the body as an assemblage of parts, or an illness as a series of discrete issues, without reference to the whole (including often vitally important emotional, psychological and spiritual issues), limits the effectiveness of much Western medicine . . .'

Iain McGilchrist, *The Master and His Emissary*

One quiet day in the late summer of 1961, my parents impulsively decided to go on a family outing. Driving in to London – a thirty-mile trip – with three young children in the back seat, we headed for the River Thames, anticipating a pleasure cruise in the tepid afternoon sun. As we arrived at the Embankment, my father parked across the road from the river. Quickly, we children tumbled out of the car in a state of excitement, hopping about to stretch our legs after the journey, as my mother opened the car boot and sorted out the cardigans and sandwiches. Looking around, I saw white buildings rise up behind us on a grand scale, shady wide pavements, the road even wider than expected, with a tantalising glimpse of the silvery river beyond. As I was taking it all in, a sudden loud and shocking screech, and then a bang, broke through the low-key murmur of London traffic, as a massive oil tanker suddenly braked in the road in front of us.

Then there was chaos. What was happening? Where was my younger sister, Vicky, then five years old? In her eagerness to see the river, she had started to cross the road – and was now lying beneath the monster truck. Lights flashed and sirens wailed as an ambulance arrived. The rest fades into a confused jumble. Vicky and my mother disappeared. At some point, my four-year-old brother and I went home with our father.

Days passed with my sister in a coma. Fragments of information were overheard. She had a fractured skull and there were fears of permanent paralysis. Would she ever come back? We were in a strange limbo.

Fortunately, she did recover, and she did come home. The doctors had saved her, and she was going to be all right. (They also saved her again, in a more low-key fashion, by administering the latest chemotherapy treatment when she got lymphoma in her fifties).

This is the most public face of health care – the accident-and-emergency services that are there when we are in extremis, saving lives at moments of crisis, such as road accidents, terrorist incidents, knifings, falls, heart attacks and respiratory failure. These are the moments of high drama when doctors' skills can often make the difference between life and death.

Popular television programmes, such as *24 Hours in A&E*, celebrate the warm humanity and skill under pressure of many of the doctors who do this work. These TV shows are never out of fashion. Throughout my childhood, the fictional *Emergency Ward 10* (with the handsome and idealistic Dr Kildare) was a favourite. Such heroic images of medicine are rooted deep in the psyche. They lie close to images of ideal parents who will protect and care for you and 'make it better'.

As a child at primary school, I enjoyed enacting these doctor-and-patient scenarios, particularly on dark, rainy days, when we couldn't go out into the playground and run around in our lunch hour. Stuck in the classroom, my best friend and I would assemble a pretend bed from a few hard upright wooden chairs and invite our classmates to take it in turns to be doctor, nurse or patient, giving imaginary injections, taking temperatures and applying bandages. As well as the frisson of touching and being touched, these games stimulated enjoyable feelings of power and authority in the caring role, and surrender to perfectly attuned carers in the patient role.

When many of my friends in adult life turned out to be health professionals, it became ever more clear to me that, while doctors and nurses care about their patients, they are highly practical people who try to fix things and rely on science to provide the tools to do so. They respond to illnesses or accidents in the here and now. However, their pressured careers offer little time to address the question of prevention, other than to pass on current received wisdom about lifestyle and the advisability of not smoking, over-eating or using mood-altering substances to excess.

A typical visit to your GP will focus on symptoms, tests and treatments. Its model of health and illness is one of a 'repair shop', where medical professionals aim to fix a body machine that is malfunctioning due to infection, dodgy genes or poor maintenance. While there is increasing awareness of how both diet and mental health play a part in illness (and vice versa), the dominant medical model, as yet, includes little recognition of the part played by stress and trauma of various kinds, particularly in early life, in creating health vulnerabilities. No GP has ever asked me about my childhood adversities, though greater awareness of their impact on my health might lead to more sensitive and effective treatment or to better screening and prevention.

A whistle-stop tour of medical history

Current attitudes to health and illness might seem 'natural', but they have emerged from a long history. Although this book will not explore it in detail, it is helpful to have in mind the rudiments of that history to appreciate why we think as we do, and what unconscious assumptions we carry about what health is and where it comes from.

Historically, our understanding of the human body was limited. Early practitioners confronted major illness with few effective weapons. Physicians and apothecaries were often overwhelmed by grave conditions they could not treat, such as dysentery, painful plagues, and mass epidemics of infectious diseases, such as cholera. There was an urgent need to find ways to treat infection effectively. However, early treatments were largely based on theories established in ancient Greece, particularly on Hippocrates's theories that health depended on maintaining a bodily balance of four 'humours' (blood, black and yellow bile, phlegm). Such theories led to the long-running practice of bloodletting, one form of which included sticking a leech on the skin of the patient to draw out an 'excess' of blood, as well as the popular practice of treating patients with toxic mercury salts to purge the body of bile.

Knowledge became more scientific when it began to be based on experiments to test new theories. However, this slow process of trial and error was often brutal, with many failures and collateral damage along the way. In the seventeenth century, for example, William Harvey's seminal discoveries about the circulation of the blood depended on cutting open live animals without benefit of anaesthetics.* Dissection of dead human bodies – another challenging practice for many medical students – also played a key role in understanding the body. It made it possible to grasp the structure of human anatomy more clearly, and to map the territory of the human body, with its organs, skeleton and muscles – a 'naming of parts'.

From time to time experiments struck lucky. The most well-known leap forward of the late eighteenth century was in fact a preventive one: vaccination against the disfiguring and often fatal

---

* The requirement to use anaesthetics and later, analgesia, in experimentation on animals was not established until the Cruelty to Animals Act of the late nineteenth century.

disease of smallpox. Although inoculation – in this case a deliberate infection with a small dose of smallpox to protect against full-blown smallpox – had been practised for centuries, particularly in North Africa and the Middle East, Edward Jenner's eighteenth-century experiment was slightly different.

Living in the Gloucestershire countryside, he noticed that the local milkmaids who had had caught cowpox, a similar but milder disease, seemed to be protected from the worst ravages of smallpox. So he set out to test this hypothesis, enlisting the eight-year-old son of his gardener as his guinea pig. He made cuts to James' arms and smeared cowpox pus into the cuts. James became unwell with cowpox symptoms for a week or two, then recovered. Jenner then proceeded to give James a small dose of smallpox itself, to see if he had developed any immunity or if he would succumb to the infection. Fortunately, the boy's body was able to mobilise the antibodies he had developed to the cowpox and he survived.

It's doubtful whether this experiment would get past a modern ethics committee, but it proved a turning point in the acceptance of vaccination by the medical profession of the time. Its success eventually enabled vaccinations to be developed for other conditions – an extraordinary step forward, which today means that many life-threatening viral illnesses, such as smallpox, polio, measles, Ebola and potentially malaria (though not a virus) – as well as Covid-19 – are on their way to being eradicated or managed.

Technological advances have also played a vital role in advancing medical knowledge. Microscopes made it possible to examine in more detail what the naked eye could not see. Their power to magnify brought various breakthroughs in the later nineteenth century, including the recognition of nerve cells as the basic units of the brain, laying the foundation for modern neuroscience. During the same era, X-ray technology was developed, revealing the current state of bones in the body, while, in the twentieth century, further technological advances in imaging, such as MRI and PET scanning, have made it possible to identify a range of biological processes inside the living body.

Getting rid of germs

By the mid-nineteenth century, scientific research was becoming established within universities. It became a more organised, sustained endeavour, which enabled scientists to work together – for example, to slowly improve and refine the technology of microscopes. Their work enabled Louis Pasteur to make the great discovery in 1860 that the active agent in many diseases is the presence of microscopic organisms called 'germs' – including bacteria and viruses – something Jenner had not known when he made his experiments. At the time, Pasteur's discovery seemed to many as implausible as science fiction – it was 'really too fantastic', according to one popular, conservative newspaper of the day.[1]

Nearly seventy years later, Alexander Fleming stumbled across a way to destroy some of these germs. In 1928, Fleming had gone on holiday, leaving an untidy lab with some staphylococcus bacteria in a small glass petri dish out on the counter. On his return, he noticed that it had gone mouldy. Examining the mould through the microscope, he saw that the 'mould juice' around the edge had actually destroyed the bacteria. Further experiments established that the mould could, in fact, kill a variety of bacteria. However, he did not follow through his discovery to experiment further, on infected mice or people. It was not until 1938 that Howard Florey (with his colleague Ernst Chain) got interested in Fleming's earlier work and began the process of refining the mould and turning it into penicillin, a highly effective treatment for infection.

Sadly, this new era of antibiotics began too late for people like my grandfather, Ben Allpress, a farmer who fell ill and developed sepsis in 1944 – a couple of years before penicillin became generally available in the UK – and he died, aged only forty. However, for the generations that followed, it has been a remarkable step forward. People living in richer countries with access to antibiotics are no longer at the mercy of many of the most dangerous bacterial infectious diseases, such as cholera, tuberculosis, and syphilis. Unfortunately, this is not the case in developing countries with fewer resources, where infectious diseases remain a major threat to health.

The drug culture

The success of antibiotics paved the way for increased financial investment in medical and scientific research in the 1950s. New technologies were developed and new drugs came on to the market: drugs to treat high blood pressure, the first anti-psychotics and tranquillisers, and the first oral hypo-glycaemic treatments for diabetes, as well as new antibiotics to deal with different infectious diseases. The market was huge and pharmaceutical companies flourished.

In the 1960s, chemotherapy was beginning to offer cures, or at least remissions, for some cancers. By the 1970s, there were new anti-inflammatories for arthritis and, in the 1980s, statins were developed – now prescribed to vast numbers of people to help prevent heart disease. Modern medicine now has a cupboard full of treatments, which are produced on an industrial scale.

The combination of aggressive marketing and wide availability has encouraged the public to turn to drugs to solve many problems. We have come to see it as normal to take pills for heartburn, colds and flu, nausea, or fever. We take pills to prevent pregnancy. We use anti-depressants to relieve distressing feelings, Ritalin to manage children's behaviour, and opioids to suppress bodily pain. Healthcare has become virtually synonymous with medication.

However, many drugs that seemed to be the solution ended up becoming part of the problem. The over-use of antibiotics has led to bacteria becoming resistant to them, leading to the threat of a new post-antibiotic era, in which common infections may kill people once again. Similarly, increasing numbers of people have become dependent on (or addicted to) strong opioid pain killers. According to the director of the US Center for Disease Control, 'America is awash with opioids'.[2] These drugs have all been developed and made available to ever-increasing numbers of people, generating vast profits. Global spending on prescription drugs is predicted to reach $1.9 trillion by 2027. Opioids alone generate around $24 billion globally, mostly in America.[3]

As medication has triumphed over many previously intractable infections, however, other dangerous conditions have taken their place as the main sources of ill health and mortality: diseases such as diabetes, cancer, cardiovascular disease and depression. These non-communicable diseases (NCDs) have shifted the focus away from infection to the 'diseases of affluence' – so-called because of their links to our changed environments, such as the rise of car ownership and air pollution, smoking, and sedentary working lives.

My genes are better than yours

While a focus on germs and ways to kill germs has become the predominant paradigm, another powerful way of thinking about health has focused on genes and how to eradicate bad genes, opening up the possibility of preventing illness before it occurs.

In the 1920s and 1930s, this became a popular movement known as eugenics. Eugenicists drew on a Mendelian* approach to genetics that assumed that genes for behaviour and health could be inherited.

---

* Mendelian genetics established that genetic traits or characteristics are passed from parents to their child. Each trait has two alleles, one from each parent. These are not blended but are either dominant or recessive. The dominant gene determines how that trait is expressed in the offspring, e.g. whether the child has brown or blue eyes.

Germs and genes

The implication was that those who were healthy (and wealthy) must have superior genes, while those who were poor or struggling were assumed to have inferior genes. What they took from genetics was the belief that even complex human traits, such as criminality, alcoholism, epilepsy or 'feeblemindedness' were controlled by single genes, which could predictably be inherited from parents.

Using charts, questionnaires and 'pedigrees', the eugenics enthusiasts graded and quantified bodily factors, such as head size and shades of skin and hair colour, itemising characteristics they deemed undesirable. In the USA, the American Eugenics Society set up stalls at local fairs, where members of the public were invited to check out their own eugenic fitness. Health, intelligence and appearance would be judged in a competition for the Fitter Family.

But the pride of the winners implied shame for the losers. One alarmist exhibit flashed a red light every forty-eight seconds to signify the frequency with which a 'feeble-minded' baby was born (while genetically fit children, apparently, were less common, and only born every seven minutes). The fittest families also appeared to be universally white . . .

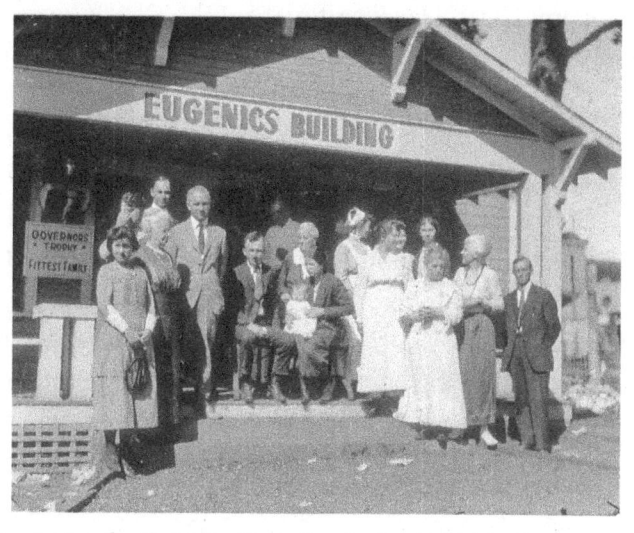

A winning family in the Fitter Family Competition, Kansas, 1925

The Eugenics movement was seen by many at the time as progressive – in Britain, its supporters included the economist John Maynard Keynes, Fabian socialists Beatrice and Sidney Webb, as well as philosopher Bertrand Russell, biologist Julian Huxley and even the mastermind of the welfare state, William Beveridge. These early twentieth-century public intellectuals were hopeful that they could create a more 'efficient' and healthy society by breeding out disabilities or undesirable traits through sterilisation. They seem, in retrospect, to have been blissfully unaware of the race, class and gender issues that were never far from the surface. An innate sense of 'us' and 'them' was at play. For example, Huxley himself suffered from severe depressions yet saw no contradiction in supporting a 1931 bill in the UK endorsing compulsory sterilisation for other people designated as 'mental patients'. Fortunately it was not passed.[4] However, in the USA, sterilisation laws *were* enacted in many states.

The harrowing life story of Carrie Buck demonstrates what this could mean in practice. She was the child of a widowed single parent accused of immorality and syphilis, who had ended up in an institution called a 'Colony' (a kind of prison for social outcasts who had not broken any laws). Her illegitimate child, Carrie, was removed from her when she was three and placed with foster parents. Although Carrie was an academically average school student, her foster parents chose to cut her education short at the age of eleven or twelve, so that she could help them with housework; by the age of seventeen, she found herself pregnant, having been raped by their nephew while her foster mother was away. Her foster parents dealt with this damage to their reputation by publicly accusing Carrie of promiscuity, calling for her to be committed to the same Colony as her mother, while taking custody of her baby for themselves.

Subsequently this vulnerable girl was chosen to be a test case for Virginia's sterilisation law, and so, in 1927, the state sought to sterilise her. Their case against her was that she was 'promiscuous'; and according to a social worker, 'obviously feebleminded'.

When the case reached the Supreme Court, Oliver Wendell Holmes, the influential judge known for his pithy opinions, pronounced: 'It is better for all the world, if instead of waiting to execute degenerate offspring for crime, or to let them starve for imbecility, society can prevent those who are manifestly unfit from continuing their kind ... Three generations of imbeciles are enough.'[5] Even into the second half of the twentieth century, forced sterilisations continued to be carried out in the USA – often on institutionalised women and women from minority ethnic groups.

However, in Europe the eugenics movement lost momentum, partly due to the uncomfortable recognition that ideas of eugenic fitness had played a major part in the Nazi regime's racist genocidal atrocities.

By the 1960s, the advent of the birth control pill had moved the goalposts. With greater control over their own fertility, women began to claim ownership of their bodies and sexual choices. It became less acceptable that the state would have a right to intervene to sterilise particular women on the grounds of their supposedly faulty genes. However, the public remained enamoured of the idea that genes accounted for individual differences in health, and hopes remained that individual genes that caused illness could be eradicated.

A fifty-year quest

The fascination with genes was given fresh impetus by the 1953 discovery of the 3D molecular structure of DNA by Crick, Watson and Franklin. This generated a new excitement about genes and renewed hopes that genes would soon provide the answer to everything: bolstered by the claim made by an exhilarated Francis Crick, when he walked into his regular pub in Cambridge, announcing: 'We have discovered the secret of life!'

This breakthrough generated a new aspiration: to map the entire human genome in the hope that it would be possible to identify the faulty genes that were the cause of disease. There were some early successes in the late 1980s and early 1990s, with the discovery of the genes for a few rare single-gene conditions, such as Huntington's disease and cystic fibrosis, which in turn generated hopes that the inherited 'genes for' many other more common diseases would soon be identified.

These were peak years for the popularity of genetic determinism, and in 1990 the Human Genome Project was launched to provide the map of all maps of human genes. A huge amount of effort and money went into this international collaboration, which finally produced its results in 2003, fifty years after the discovery of the structure of DNA. The project's achievements in developing sequencing technologies were impressive. However, it did not result in startling new discoveries of 'genes for' particular illnesses, as was hoped. Instead, it became clear that it is rare for a mutation in a single gene to cause a disease.

As geneticists revised their expectations, they redirected scientific attention towards understanding how networks of thousands of genes might operate together to create complex traits or illnesses. From around 2005, these 'genome-wide association studies' (GWAS) took off, again hoping to find the genes associated with particular illnesses. Although GWAS studies have succeeded in finding common genetic variants associated with some complex diseases, such huge numbers of genes are involved that these explain only a small percentage of disease risk. Even when combining all available GWAS on a particular disorder, polymorphisms usually explain less than 5%–10% of the risk of disease. The discovery that having the genetic mutation BRCA1 or BRCA2 significantly increases the risk of developing breast cancer, for example, does not mean that it is the sole cause of breast cancer: in fact, these inherited genes are responsible for only 5%–10% of all breast cancers.[6]

Critics such as the journalist Nicholas Wade have argued that these genome-wide association studies have not as yet been that useful clinically. In an article for the *New York Times*, he wrote: 'One sign of the genome's limited use for medicine so far was a recent test of genetic predictions for heart disease. A medical team led by Nina P. Paynter of Brigham and Women's Hospital in Boston collected 101 genetic variants that had been statistically linked to heart disease in various genome-scanning studies. But the variants turned out to have no value in forecasting disease among 19,000 women who had been followed for 12 years'.[7] Attempts to find the genes associated with educational attainment also fell flat in a big 2013 study of 127,000 people, which found that genes were responsible for 'a mere 0.02 per cent of the difference in attainment – about 1 month of schooling'.[8]

Despite such disappointments, the strong public belief in genetic determinism remains largely unshaken. A commonly held view persists that genes are an instruction manual that dictates how a person will develop, according to a pre-ordained plan. The mass media and the public often continue to think in a simplistic way about genes 'for' particular traits and genes 'causing' behaviours or illnesses.[9]

The poster boy for such hard-line genetic determinism has for decades been the influential behavioural geneticist Robert Plomin, rated as 'one of the top 100 most eminent psychologists of the twentieth century'.[10] Recorded online in his light-filled, art-adorned university study, he continues, in the twenty-first century, to insist that genes are 'the most important factor shaping who we are' – the 'blueprint for who we are'.[11] Rather than understanding each of us as adaptable individuals with multiple potentials, which unfold only in a particular social and ecological context, Plomin dismisses the effects of the environment as a 'temporary' influence; once it passes, the individual will return to his or her genetic trajectory.[12] Plomin's views fit well with an individualistic culture and individualistic medicine that understands people as the possessors of a unique set of genes, which determine how intelligent, how healthy or even how kind they are. For Plomin, differences in parenting are irrelevant:

'Nice parents have nice children because they are all nice genetically'.[13]

Despite his calm, unruffled persona, Plomin has always seemed to enjoy provoking and challenging those who give weight to the nurture side of the nature versus nurture debate. In 1984, he scoffed that such 'environmentalists' are reduced to clutching at straws – their 'last resort', as he put it, is to attribute differences in personality to 'the perinatal and prenatal periods. If these early environments could be shown to influence personality, the extreme environmental position would be tenable and there could be a continued denial of genetic causation'.[14] The evidence presented in this book suggests that this 'extreme environmental position' is not so extreme.

For a growing number of scientists, there has been a rapprochement between the previously antagonistic nature and nurture camps, and the emergence of a friendly new consensus that it is 'a bit of both' – that genes and environment interact and affect each other. Most geneticists are now more likely to talk of polygenic and multifactorial causes of illness. The language has become more nuanced. One panel of experts described inherited genetic variation within families as a 'contribution' to the 'pathogenesis of disease', that might lead to a 'susceptibility to particular diseases'.[15] Others have described the new genomics as 'a transformed enterprise that also focuses on data about proteins, DNA methylation patterns or the physiology and the environment of the people studied; DNA sequence data now forms only part of a much larger picture'.[16]

Epigenetics

The growing field of 'epigenetics', in particular, has given fresh impetus to the environmental/nurture side of the equation. The timing was serendipitous. Just as the work of the Human Genome

Project was drawing to a close, this emerging body of work started to gather momentum. As the Californian psychologist David Moore describes, in his book *The Developing Genome*,[17] his online PubMed search for 'epigenetics' in 1999 turned up only forty-six references. By 2013, PubMed found 2,413 papers that mentioned it.

Epigenetics changes the way we think about genes. It has made it clear that genes are much more interactive than previously thought. Like the ingredients in a store cupboard, genes contain information that can be used or 'expressed' by being translated into proteins – or can be left in the gene cupboard unused. Being the owner of particular genes is not a reliable guide as to whether or not they will be expressed in that person's lifetime. Genes themselves don't dictate which protein to make – the information stored in genes is 'expressed' when needed by events within the body or demands from the external environment. These pressures, including emotional and social experiences, trigger biochemical reactions.

Epigenetic processes are one way of affecting gene expression. In the epigenetic process, certain biochemicals become attached to genes and either *prevent* them from expressing certain characteristics (in the process of DNA methylation, which has been described as a 'protective cover' on the DNA) or can *activate* gene expression (through histone acetylation of DNA). As Gertrudis Van de Vijver and her colleagues at Ghent University put it: 'Instead of containing the core program or the basic instructions of the living, the genome is viewed as a regulatory system that actively responds to internal and external fluctuations of various kinds'.[18] For example, a child may respond to high levels of stress by methylating, or covering, the glucocorticoid receptor (GR) genes that are involved in managing stress. When the expression of these genes is prevented by methylation, the outcome can be a tendency to develop an exaggerated or hypersensitive response to stress, lasting, in some cases, for a lifetime.[19] Conversely, soothing activities, such as breastfeeding and gentle stroking in the early months of life, can increase the expression of GR genes and reduce the child's reactivity to stress.[20]

Epigenetic 'marks' on the genes are, in effect, a way that cells remember an environmental factor, in order to anticipate the future and prepare for it. In some cases, these epigenetic alterations can even be passed on down the generations. However, some epigenetic effects are also flexible enough to be reversible when the environment changes. For example, experiments with rats have shown that improving their diets by giving them methionine (an amino acid found in foods such as eggs, meat and seafood) can reverse the epigenetic marks that altered their stress responses as infants.[21] Similarly, improved nutrition may influence the course of cancer. Cancer is thought to start with genetic variants or epigenetic changes that can activate cancer genes (oncogenes) or silence the genes responsible for suppressing tumours. There is some (as yet inconclusive) evidence to suggest that the abnormal epigenetic alterations involved in cancer may be affected by plant foods containing phytochemicals (such as particular vegetables and fruits, herbs, spices and beans). Phytochemicals may help to repress cancer-related genes and re-activate the tumour suppression genes.[22] Hearteningly, it is also possible for the epigenetic alterations and premature biological ageing linked to early childhood adversities to be reversed to some extent if the individual's social status improves.[23]

Many psychologists, neuroscientists, ecologists, biologists and paediatricians now concur with epigeneticists that each person's unique characteristics – his or her individual 'phenotype' – comes from the interaction between their personal genome and their unique environment, starting even in the womb.[24] There is a complex interplay between our bodies, our biology and our social experience. However, this complexity is more difficult to present to the public than a model that suggests there is a 'gene for' everything.

An individual's genes play a part in our life, not because they drive events but because they respond and adapt to events: 'Phenotypes... are not determined by what is inside or outside but rather by how the inside and the outside influence one another.'[25] As David Moore put it, 'If we want to know whether a baby is going to be exceptionally bright as an adult, we're going to have to wait to find out'.[26]

This new understanding is tipping the old nature–nurture debate away from the concept of an individual 'battle' with risky genes or threatening pathogens, supported by medical troops on the hospital and pharmaceutical 'frontline', to wider questions of how to create an environment that supports health. The unconscious bias of medical thinking has been an individualistic framework: how to fix it? What is the cure? The question that seems to be rarely asked is why people get diabetes, arthritis or depression, or how we can ensure the development of an effective immune system to prevent illness in the first place, or how we might balance out a predisposition to certain health conditions.

What if we shift our focus to include the importance of achieving health as well as battling illness? We might need to give greater consideration to the sources of good health: how the food we eat affects our bodies, how health falters when people's psychological resources fail them or when stresses of life overwhelm them. Recognising our vulnerabilities rather than simply trying to muster our warrior intentions would enable us to see more clearly the role of good food, good relationships and good environments in creating health – and would encourage us to value everyday 'care', both at home and in our social institutions.

Hi-tech or low

Today, however, mainstream medicine is still dominated by 'heroic' thinking, particularly in the pursuit of new technologies and the building of ever more space-age mega-hospitals. 'Care' is the shabby old relative who rarely gets invited to the party.

It's easy to see the appeal of high-tech approaches when technology has achieved so much to improve health outcomes. Particularly for policy-makers and managers of health care, faced with the choice between spending money on a dissolvable stent instead of a metal one for coronary artery blockage, or spending it on support groups for pregnant women, the high-tech option might look more like 'real' medicine. It is also the option that will be supported by the large companies who can make money out of it. Their influence can be seen in government policy choices. In practice, governments work hand in hand with business, funding and encouraging such ventures. In the UK, for instance, ministers for 'life sciences' have sometimes been appointed with the job of transforming the British National Health Service through health technology and innovation. One former life sciences minister, George Freeman, depicts himself as a lover of nature who enjoys walking across the flat fields of his unspoilt rural constituency of Norfolk in his spare time. As a politician, however, he pursued what he perceived as 'cutting-edge' new technology, drawing on his previous career as a biomedical venture capitalist to enthuse the public about turning the health service into a platform for biotech and genomics entrepreneurs. Speaking with animation at Imperial College in London in 2016, he launched his strategic plan for the 'bio-economy'. His ambition was to make health care 'the booming industry of the twenty-first century'. In the USA, too, these technological innovations are seen as a vital driver of economic growth.[27]

In January 2016, this had been a key idea at the World Economic Forum in Davos; political and business leaders, such as the Russian-born co-founder of Google, Sergey Brin, were gripped with excitement at the prospect of a Fourth Industrial Revolution based on new technologies, heralding an era of 'revolutionary change in the way the railway age did for the Victorians'. Newly developing technologies would bring jobs, companies, and fresh opportunities. The hot game in town seemed to be the prospect of making money out of science, or of 'commercialising science into economic value', as George Freeman put it in a speech a few weeks after Davos. He took up the baton of this new 'age of biology', describing how entrepreneurs could make use of 'the intracellular journey of understanding the causal mechanisms of disease [. . .] using the cells as the factories of the twenty-first century'.[28]

This latest vision of medical progress through technology may be cutting edge, but it fits seamlessly into a narrative of health that has been running since the actual industrial revolution of the early nineteenth century. At the heart of the narrative is a belief that pioneering individuals can conquer nature, and make a profit doing so. The public, in turn, trusts that these medical pioneers will come up with fixes to halt disease in its tracks and postpone death.

Freeman argued that the technologies he champions are the way forward to create more efficient health services. For example, the 'translational medicine' approach encourages researchers to collaborate across disciplines and with industry to apply new research findings as rapidly as possible in clinical settings, giving patients access to new drugs more quickly.

'Informatics' is about storing data and using it to feed into research or into individual patient care. Despite problems with confidentiality and with cybersecurity, this now seems unstoppable. Progress in informatics can bring cheap and efficient devices that collect health data, such as a portable electroencephalogram (EEG) monitor, or an app that connects to an EEG headset, which researchers can use to study people's brains in natural settings, or a watch that continuously monitors glucose levels for diabetics. Data can now be stored and passed on rapidly through smart phones and could improve healthcare productivity by keeping people out of hospital and enabling earlier diagnosis via video calls with doctors, or by offering mental health treatments, such as cognitive behaviour therapy (CBT), digitally. Under pressure from Covid-19 restrictions, many of these have already been adopted.

Personalised medicine or genomics is about using drugs more effectively. It uses genetic data to tailor treatments or to adjust doses to ensure that pharmaceutical drugs are used only when likely to be effective for that particular individual (currently, many medications are more miss than hit). In cancer treatment, genomics are starting to be used to identify tumours with specific genetic characteristics; these can be identified by a diagnostic test, and then targeted with the drugs most likely to be effective, based on the patient's own personal sensitivity and resistance. It can also be used to identify new uses for old drugs, or new niche populations that could benefit from specific drugs.

Many of these innovations could potentially help to make health services more streamlined and cost-effective. Like watching the heroes of a fast-paced action movie, there are always exciting new possibilities to explore when it comes to health technologies. Nevertheless, set in the context of cash-starved public health services, and a healthcare system in crisis, they may seem crazily beside the point. We fail to provide good care for our elder generation, yet we can genetically modify embryos. Current policies do not adequately address the key challenges faced by Western health systems in the twenty-first century: the expansion of the ageing population, unremitting health inequalities, and the financial burden of dramatic rises in chronic conditions, such as obesity, diabetes and dementia. In the USA, Alzheimer's disease alone is seen by some as 'a disease on track to bankrupt Medicare'.[29] Making medications more accurate or more focused on those patients who can benefit from them, or managing chronic illnesses more effectively, does not tackle their underlying root causes. Today, what would be truly revolutionary would be to understand enough to prevent these conditions in the first place.

But followers of the capitalist way are selective about the science that interests them. They prefer the clear-cut solutions offered by technology, following the Enlightenment model: drugs and hard data, with commercial possibilities, treatments that will generate wealth and power, solutions that will make us feel more in control.

They are not often, if ever, heard enthusing about the other revolution that is brewing in public health: the 'soft' stuff of understanding the early developmental origins of ill health in pregnancy and infancy, the science of early nurture and nutrition, and the interactive nature of body and brain development. One reason for this is that these un-heroic activities offer few commercial opportunities. How can money be made by encouraging the consumption of unprocessed food or in supporting warm relationships?

Low tech

Yet a voluminous, ever-expanding body of scientific work consistently points us to these 'low-tech' solutions to many of our mental and physical health problems. This work has primarily emerged in the period since the Second World War. Its findings were not available when the British NHS was established, and health services around the world have taken relatively little notice of them since.

The key sources of the low-tech science revolution lie in developmental psychology, neuroscience, nutritional research, bacteriology, and epidemiology. Cumulatively, these late twentieth-century disciplines are becoming more integrated, offering a fresh framework for understanding mental and physical health. Together, these newly flourishing disciplines enlarge our concepts of health and illness beyond the individual body, to the ways that the individual body is embedded in the social world. Moving away from the dominant model focused on fixing ill health that is primarily caused by our enemies (i.e. bad genes, accidents or bad infectious agents), the developmental perspective has shown how much good health depends on positive interactions with other people and on good food and uncontaminated physical environments, particularly in early life.

This perspective offers the hope of collective solutions to health issues and to the possibilities of preventing both mental and physical ill health, if only we are able to look at long-term solutions and not just instant cures for the current ailment. But to get behind such an approach, both governments and voters need a much clearer vision of the underlying causes of our chronic health problems – a new story that can help us understand how people are grown and how to grow healthier people.

2.

Growing a person:
a social, interactive view of health

'It's like every new person is a completely new roll of the dice, right?'

Marilynne Robinson, *New York Review of Books*

During my daughter's pregnancy, we awaited the new baby with keen anticipation and wondered what kind of person they would be. An ultrasound scan revealed my future grandson had long legs, so we started to speculate: will he be tall? Athletic? Talkative? Who will he take after? Although he represents a fresh genetic 'roll of the dice', with all its possibilities and hindrances, I am also aware that, in practice, much of any new person's potential only emerges in response to the relationships and environmental resources available to them.

This is a very different understanding from the dominant Western ideology of individualism, whose assumptions were indirectly revealed by the novelist Marilynne Robinson in a discussion she had with Barack Obama a few years ago. She exclaimed rhetorically, 'What does freedom mean? I mean, really, the ideal of freedom if it doesn't mean that we can find out what is in this completely unique being that each one of us is?'[1] Her words implied that each person has a unique future self already there 'in' each one of us, waiting to be found, as long as there are no obstacles to our freedom and agency.

What this commonly held view leaves out is that, as well as our genes, there is another roll of the dice that matters – our given social, familial and physical environment. The social world of our early years and the environment in which we live can have a biological impact on our body and lasting health. As the American sociologist Charles Cooley put it over a century ago: 'A separate individual is an abstraction unknown to experience ...'[2] Yet the important developmental and environmental story has often been side-lined. It has been waiting in the wings for much of the last century, making repeated guest appearances, but never becoming the main attraction – till now.

Social influences on health

Many currents of thought contributed to the emergence of a more social and developmental perspective on health in the later nineteenth and early twentieth centuries. One factor was a growing public awareness of the disastrous consequences of external circumstances – in this case, industrialisation – on the health of the poorer sectors of society. In the UK, two reports on the living conditions of the urban poor – one by the public health reformer Edwin Chadwick and another by the political activist Friedrich Engels – had been published in the 1840s. They described overcrowded, ramshackle housing that often lacked clean water and sanitation; and how, as a result, infectious diseases were rife. A shocking number of babies (as high as 20% in some areas) did not survive their first year. Nutrition was minimal. One 1892 study reported that, even at the end of the century, 'the poor children of Bethnal Green were nourished almost entirely on bread'.[3] As British Army recruiters discovered in the early twentieth century, these inadequate living conditions meant that large numbers of potential young soldiers had suffered serious childhood illnesses, rickets and malnutrition and were in such poor physical condition that they were unfit for combat.

Projects to build social infrastructure gathered momentum. There was a successful drive to improve the water supply and to expand the public sewers, measures that helped to bring down the number of infant deaths. Concerned bodies sent in 'sanitary visitors' to the homes of the poor, offering advice on hygiene and instruction on the care and feeding of babies. By 1929, this had culminated in a new profession of health visitors, which may have contributed to a dramatic fall in infant mortality.[4]

As the twentieth century began, new disciplines, such as neuroscience and psychology, were emerging, as well as a renewal of Mendelian genetics. Interest in child development increased. Inspired by Charles Darwin's theories of evolution, the child study movement led by Stanley Hall tried to understand how children's behaviour developed as an adaptive response to the world around them. At the same time, some exciting but speculative theories, such as the psychoanalytic work of Sigmund Freud, Anna Freud and Melanie Klein, generated interest in children's earliest emotions and unconscious processes. All hoped and believed that greater scientific understanding would be able to deliver better child health and solve social problems.

By the 1920s, dubbed the 'Decade of the Child', a growing band of professional child experts set out to apply the scientific method of systematic observation, experimentation and testing to map out the processes of 'normal' mental and physical development, much in the same way that early medical scientists had mapped out the human body and its organs. Like the eugenicists of the same period, their focus was on the individual child and on what could be observed and measured in the laboratory: the child's weight and height, stages of development, milestones, personality type, motor and cognitive development or predictable responses to stimuli. Lacking modern technical resources, such as PET scans, videos or computational statistics – which can highlight more dynamic and interactive aspects of child health – they relied on external observation to pin down the fixed 'laws' of nature or personal traits as they developed.

Wealthy US philanthropists, such as the Rockefeller family, supported these scientific endeavours by pouring serious money (obtained from the growing profitability of industrial mass production and from a booming oil business) into new child study institutes. With reliable long-term funding, some of these institutes were able to set up the first studies that followed people from babyhood over many years, in order to establish how their development unfolded at different ages. One of the first of these early 'birth cohort' studies was the Berkeley Guidance Study, which studied a group of babies born in 1928 through to adulthood in 1946. These cohort studies were to bear fruit over the long term, as researchers began to interpret the data afresh, particularly in relation to social change and historic events such as the Great Depression and the Second World War.

By 1930, this growing interest in children's welfare reached a high point when US President Herbert Hoover convened a conference on child health, endorsing its importance while stating: 'If we could have one generation of properly born, trained, educated and healthy children, a thousand other problems of government would vanish'.[5]

Seeing the child in context

In those decades, child 'training' – focused on authority and discipline – was the main way that people thought of 'parenting'. In the early twentieth century, a campaigner for better infant health called Dr Truby King argued that it was essential to train children from infancy into good 'habits'. He defined these as strictly regular times for babies' feeding, bowel movements 'by the clock', and even a rejection of the 'fond and foolish overindulgence' of warm physical contact, such as co-sleeping or cuddling. Paradoxically, new, more child-centred, ways of thinking were also emerging; they saw the goal of parenting in a different light. In particular, the child guidance movement of the 1920s and 1930s was influential. Partly derived from Freudian thinking, which was becoming increasingly fashionable during these decades – at least at the dinner tables of the chattering classes – child guidance clinics took a surprisingly social view of child health and development. Their new psychology argued for the importance of meeting children's emotional needs to support their development. Their underlying assumption was that the child was an 'adaptive social being' whose development was influenced by interacting with his or her circumstances.[6]

In the UK, one person who was influenced by such thinking was John Bowlby, the British physician and psychoanalyst, who had himself worked in a child guidance clinic at the end of the 1930s. He drew on these experiences to write a report pointing out that many children who were labelled 'maladjusted' had suffered separation from their mothers in early life, or had hostile fathers. He believed their anti-social behaviour could be better understood by understanding their relationship experiences.[7] Bowlby became a key figure in shifting study of the child away from innate capacities, such as intelligence or sexual drives, and instead focusing on understanding the child in the context of the parent/child relationship. By the 1950s, his 'attachment theory' was taking shape. As a scientist, Bowlby was interested in the biological purpose of early attachment relationships. He recognised that the child's biological needs could only be met through a caregiver, and he saw that the infant's need to form an early attachment relationship was driven by the child's biological instinct for survival. Importantly, Bowlby also had an American collaborator, the psychologist Mary Ainsworth, who devised a way of scientifically assessing the nature and quality of this early attachment relationship. Known as the Strange Situation test, which observed how a toddler reacted to a short separation from the parent, this experimental procedure enabled attachment research to take off in universities in the USA, under the umbrella of developmental psychology. By the 1970s, its influence was spreading as empirical data kept confirming the tenets of attachment theory.[8]

Another psychologist, Urie Bronfenbrenner, argued for a wider scope of social influences on child development. A pioneer of the Head Start programme of early intervention in the USA, his 'ecological systems theory' argued that children were 'biopsychosocial' systems who not only interacted with their family and neighbourhood, but also with wider socio-economic systems, including government and the wider culture. As he described it, humans develop through their reciprocal interactions both with the people around them and also with their wider cultural and physical environment, in a process that gets more and more complex as it goes on.[9]

This new developmental and systemic thinking motivated other psychologists to set up fresh birth cohort studies in the early 1970s. The Minnesota study was focused on a small group of babies who started life in poverty, and its aim was to explore the longer-term effects of their early attachment experiences. The Dunedin study in New Zealand had a different focus. It recruited a larger group of around 1,000 urban, relatively 'socio-economically advantaged' babies born over the course of one year, with the aim of assessing their health and development at the age of three, in relation to their social and family experiences. Interestingly, early results at three years old revealed that around 10% of parents had difficulty managing and controlling their toddlers, or had issues with their children's eating, sleeping, or ability to separate from their mother – and around 25% of children showed some degree of developmental delay in speaking or walking.[10] These results invited further investigation. As it turned out, both studies proved to be seminal and long-lasting, continuing to follow 'their' children over many decades.

Homing in on the developmental process

The developmental view emphasised the way that we grow through a ceaseless process of interaction with the world around us, right from the very start of life. But our life experiences are not automatically laid down in our brains 'like a tape recorder with the record button always on', with new experiences writing over and replacing earlier experiences.[11] Some experiences leave more of a trace than others. Intense or repeated experiences register as memories in neural networks. Some experiences leave their 'mark' on the genes; others don't. Different kinds of learning create structure and pattern in our brains, physiology and personalities. How we experience the present depends on both the mental and physiological structures formed by past experience. We learn, we remember, the past interacts with the present, we get more complex, we develop.

Our history plays a much bigger role in our development than we have allowed. 'It is never just genes and environment but always genes, environment, and history that determine growth', as Alan Sroufe, the calmly-spoken attachment-based psychologist behind the Minnesota project, put it, with his usual lucidity. Every living plant, animal or human has a story – how they respond to circumstances, how they evolve or adapt over time, and how earlier developmental choices influence later ones. In my recent attempts to grow small tangy tomatoes, I note that some of the seedlings flourish, while others die prematurely. Plants that were poorly supported as they grew may bend in a certain direction, and snap in a storm. Those planted in the cooler shade may grow short, yet produce the green tomatoes I want for my favourite chutney. Even snowflakes have a history: though each one is formed from the same elements, each crystal takes a unique form depending on chance elements of its existence.[12]

The lives of animals and humans are also subject to chance. We have no control over our genetic 'roll of the dice' nor the environment we find ourselves in as children. Yet so much of the development of our genetic potentials depends on the nurture we receive and the stresses we endure, particularly in our early lives.

Our very earliest experiences matter so much partly because development is a cumulative process. It is always constrained by what has gone before. These early experiences set us off in a

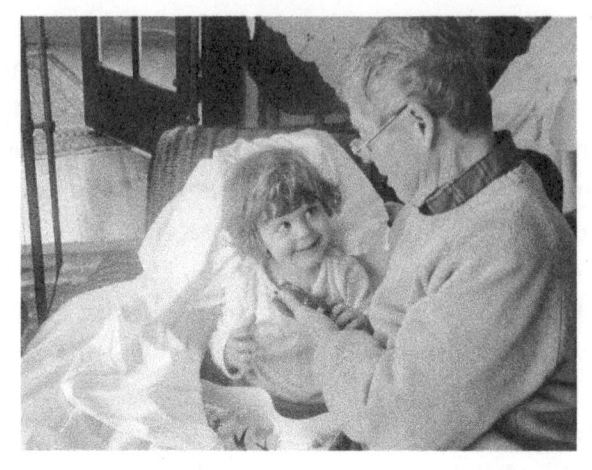

American developmental psychologist Professor Alan Sroufe with his granddaughter

direction of travel. They furnish us with basic expectations and models of reality, as well as organising our physiological systems in particular ways. Some of these events are hard to modify at a later date. Yet, at the same time, there are still many opportunities throughout our life to reorganise and to build new structures, based on repeated new experiences.

Timing and sensitive periods

Timing can be crucial. 'Developmental time is not uniform in its potency and influence'[13] – some periods are more 'plastic' and open to change than others. The most crucial moments are when a structure, system or body part is forming. Alan Sroufe describes a rather horrible experiment with chick embryos. As he explains, at the moment of development when leg and wing buds are just emerging, you can move a piece of leg tissue and put it at the tip of the wing, and it will become an integral part of the wing. However, if you do this transfer slightly later in development, it will not take, because the tissue is already 'committed' to becoming leg tissue. At some intermediate point between the two, 'the tissue becomes neither normal wing nor anomalous leg tissue, but a claw!'[14] As he puts it, the timing can be 'exquisite'.

In human development, timing matters too. The whole period from conception through to the end of the second year, approximately the first 1,001 days, is full of moments such as these.

Much has been made of whether these are critical periods or merely sensitive periods. The distinction is about whether developmental events are 'now or never', and whether, if things go wrong in an important period of development, this is likely to be irreversible. As we will explore in the next chapters, there are some changes in the embryo and fetus that may indeed be so. But there are also more flexible and less well-defined periods of development that merely have a strong influence on our lives.

The sensitive body

Sensitive periods are currently defined as 'periods of heightened plasticity, during which the development of both brain and behaviour are highly receptive to particular experiential information'.[15] There is a scientific consensus that early life has a particular impact, and that 'exposures occurring very early in development may have more pronounced effects on development than those that occur later'.[16] There are many overlapping sensitive periods that can have long-term effects on the brain and the body, but the general principle is that a sensitive period occurs when systems are being set up or being reorganised.

This starts in the womb, when the basic structures of the body are being assembled. The nutrition the fetus gets can affect the basic size of organs, the number of fat cells, as well as the number of neurons that form the brain's grey matter – in effect, its 'hardware'. The post-natal period, on the other hand, is when much of the 'software' is established. This refers to the connecting systems that communicate between organs and the brain, using neurotransmitters, hormones and their receptors. Most notably, this is when the body's regulatory systems mature. These will be explored further in subsequent chapters, but include our stress response, as well as the vagal nerve system, the immune system and the gut microbiome – none of which are fully functional at birth. Once a system is well established, it should be able to deal effectively with a challenge or disturbance and find its way back to a state of equilibrium: 'As a sensitive period closes, the organisation of neural circuits becomes increasingly stable.'[17]

Infancy is not the only sensitive period. Other key moments for new learning and brain re-organisation are early adolescence, and old age. Nevertheless, along with pre-natal development, infancy is the period of most rapid and dramatic brain growth and physiological organisation, which has huge significance for our direction of travel in life. The way that the brain and body systems are structured in this stage becomes the scaffolding on which later experience can be built.

Questions about sensitive periods

A common rebuttal to the concept of sensitive periods is that since we go on learning and making new connections between neurons in the brain throughout life, early development is not definitive. This argument, made by the contrarians at the Centre for Parenting Culture Studies, draws heavily on the work of the cognitive scientist John Bruer. At their conference in 2014, Bruer (whose book was first published in 1999) repeated arguments based on the old-fashioned notion that child development is largely about cognition. Bruer denies the importance of social and emotional development in the first 1,000 days, arguing that as long as vision, hearing or language problems are fixed early, then what matters to Bruer – 'learning to read, and subsequent educational success' – will be unaffected. For him, projects to support under three-year-olds, such as Head Start in the USA, are a waste of resources.[18]

Bruer's thinking remains stuck in the old seventeenth-century Enlightenment paradigm that separates body and mind, keeping the mechanical body and its brain apart. New developmental thinking, on the other hand, recognises that bodies, emotions and brains are interconnected systems. The capacity to regulate these systems is every bit as important as reading and is first learnt in infancy. Ironically, self-regulation even underpins the capacity to pay attention and thus has a huge impact on learning. In fact, early cognitive learning itself depends on relationship experiences. For example, our verbal development as babies relies not only on hearing people talking around us, but on our parents talking *to* us,[19] and especially on parents interpreting and naming our feelings and emotions.[20]

Learning to regulate the body

During early life, our body is being 'programmed' by experience to manage itself in various ways. In particular, physiological systems are organising themselves around 'set points'. The body tries to find stability (or 'homeostasis') by keeping systems operating within a certain normal range based around a set point. This is achieved by constant monitoring of the cellular environment. The set points are adaptable; they respond to feedback from the environment and can be re-set if conditions change over time. Some set points are tightly fixed, while others are loosely controlled and have more leeway. For example, body temperature can fluctuate, generating a high temperature or even fever when needed, but will then return to the set point of 37 degrees. Body weight is also adjustable; the body tolerates quite a wide range of weights, – one reason why it is so easy to get stuck at the overweight end of the scale.[21] However, this early physiological regulation depends on other people. For example, a newborn baby cannot manage his or her body temperature without an adult to keep him or her warm or cool him or her down, nor can he or she satisfy his or her hunger and grow without an adult to provide milk.

The body's regulatory systems themselves can also be affected by the *quality* of the early relationship. In particular, a stressful attachment relationship can undermine the effectiveness of the defensive stress and immune systems, while a secure attachment supports soothing and calming systems, such as the oxytocin system and the vagal system (both explored in more detail in Chapter Five). Those of us who benefited from relaxed, safe social attachments with supportive parents are likely to be able to recover more quickly from stress and inflammation, while those who did not enjoy an emotionally available and responsive early relationship may be at greater risk of developing a dysregulated stress response with less ability to switch off inflammation, increasing the risk of future inflammation-based illnesses.

Using the brain to regulate

Another seminal figure who emerged in the 1980s and 1990s was Allan Schore, sometimes referred to as 'the American Bowlby'. An intense, voluble New Yorker, he worked tirelessly through the 1980s as an independent researcher seeking to understand links between the new fields of affective neuroscience (the neuroscience of emotion), developmental psychology and psychoanalysis. He amassed a vast quantity of research and finally published his first magisterial volume in the early 1990s – one of many thick tomes that clarified the underlying biology of the developmental process.

Schore homed in on the importance of long-underestimated, largely mammalian forms of emotional communication between people. Eye contact, touch and vocal intonation are meaningful throughout life, but vital for survival and development when we are infants. While the psychologist Steven Porges focused on how these forms of connection in early life affected the vagal nerve, Schore

Growing a person: a social, interactive view of health

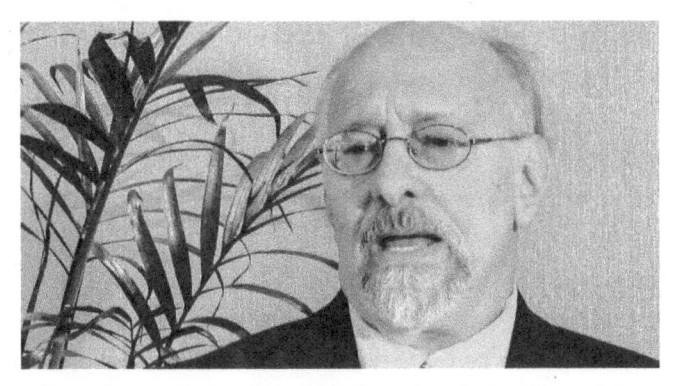

Dr Allan Schore, whose ground-breaking 'regulation theory' showed how early relationships affect the development of the brain and body

explained how they could also shape certain circuits in our developing brain. He found that positive social relationships in infancy strengthen neural connections in the parts of the brain colloquially called the 'social brain' (particularly the medial prefrontal cortex), which plays an important role in managing and regulating emotions triggered by the amygdala. Schore described just how interactive this process is. As he put it, 'the self-organisation of the developing brain occurs in the context of a relationship with another self, another brain', via the largely non-verbal communication taking place between a parent's right brain and a baby's right brain during the early months when attachment relationships are being forged.[22] Over twenty years later, there is an overwhelming consensus among researchers in the field that 'variation in early-life experience can persistently alter the development and function of these circuits'.[23]

Schore's 'regulation theory' outlined how early attachment figures help us modulate our emotions as children – to make them stronger or weaker, to hold them back or express them. Yet a surprising number of us don't realise what a crucial role our parents (and other caregivers) played in cultivating these social and emotional skills. In the USA, one large survey found that even in the twenty-first century, as many as 36% of parents expected babies under the age of two to know automatically how to control their emotions and thought their babies and toddlers should be punished for bad behaviour.[24] One third of American families also reported spanking children as young as ten to eighteen months of age.[25] Although smacking children today seems to be in decline and is outlawed in several countries, a more recent study of parents' spanking behaviour worldwide found that 63% of two- to four-year-olds were regularly physically punished.[26] It seems that the 'training' model of parenting still prevails for many adults.

In fact, the best way for toddlers to learn self-control is to watch adults modelling such behaviour, and the surest path to developing empathy for others is being on the receiving end of empathy. The most self-aware adults are often those who had parents who helped them to become aware by noticing and talking about their feelings from an early age; being able to put feelings into words can play a helpful part in managing and controlling them.

However, when parental figures are not so helpful at supporting emotional regulation, or worse, when their own behaviour consistently increases a child's stress, this too can have consequences for physiological development.

How the body copes with stress

The late 1980s and 1990s were a fertile time for developmental psychology and neuroscience. There was a blossoming of interdisciplinary networks of scientists who shared their findings and sometimes worked together. One benefit of this blending of psychology and biology was that it brought greater awareness of the impact that psychological stresses in early life could have on the body's regulatory systems.

The work of notable developmental psychobiologists, such as Megan Gunnar, homed in on one of these systems – the stress response. In 1985, it had become possible to measure the level of the stress hormone cortisol in saliva, enabling researchers to test cortisol

Growing a person: a social, interactive view of health

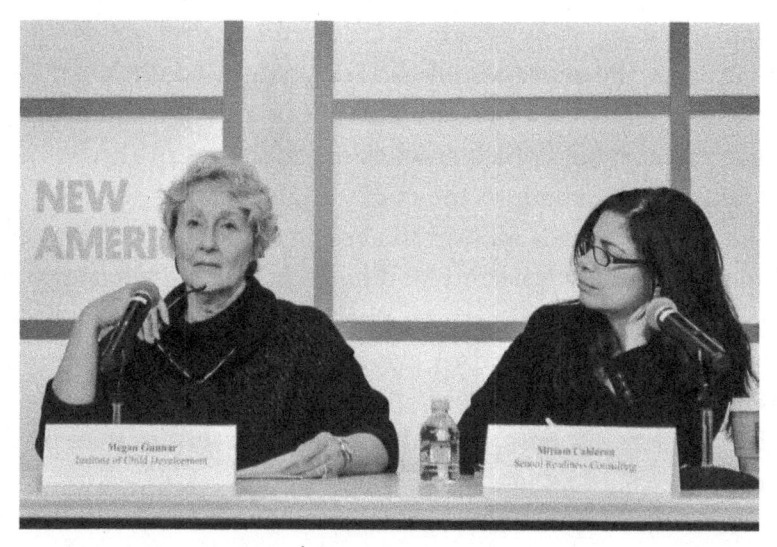

Professor Megan Gunnar with a colleague. Gunnar's work has explored how early life adversity can shape stress reactivity and regulation

levels with greater ease. This allowed Gunnar and her colleagues to explore how early stress could affect a child's stress response.[27]

The stress response

A crucial aspect of survival is our ability to deal with threats to our well-being, whether they come from the physical environment, such as a speeding car, or from other people when they treat us badly. The body's first line of defence against such challenges is known as 'fight or flight': this is when the sympathetic nervous system quickly releases adrenaline and noradrenaline, increasing the heart rate and blood pressure so the individual can more effectively either fight or run away from danger.*

If the stressful situation persists, the rapid response of the

---

* If neither option is possible, the last resort is to 'freeze' as a mouse does when it plays dead in the jaws of a cat – a state activated by the lower vagal nerve.

sympathetic nervous system is followed up, after about fifteen minutes, by the activation of the HPA axis (Hypothalamic Pituitary Adrenal) stress response. This releases an extra burst of the hormone cortisol, which reaches many tissues in the body by 'binding' or attaching to the cortisol (glucocorticoid) receptors (GRs) found on cells all over the body and brain. The extra cortisol triggers the release of blood sugar, which helps generate the energy needed to deal with an ongoing stressor for a few hours. At the same time, cortisol also dampens down the immune system, temporarily stopping immune cells from launching an inflammatory response, so the body can focus its resources on the most immediate threat.

Normally, once the cells are filled up with cortisol, cortisol receptors in the brain's hypothalamus perceive that extra cortisol is no longer needed, and stop producing it – a process known as 'negative feedback'.[28] The production of cortisol can then return to its normal daily rhythm, which is a peak of cortisol in the early morning as the individual meets the day with fresh energy, followed by pulses of cortisol to renew energy through the day. The immune system can also resume its normal operations.

The stress system works well as a brief turbo-charged reaction to deal with short-term challenges. However, some threats are not short term, particularly those involving psychological conflict or unsafe environments. When people have to deal with chronic – or particularly severe – stress, the system may not work so well. Eventually the body adjusts to the ongoing release of cortisol by switching off the cortisol receptor genes themselves (in an epigenetic process described in Chapter One). However, this can undermine the negative feedback process.[29]

The developing stress system of a fetus can be affected by the stresses faced by its mother. Particularly from mid-pregnancy on, a highly stressed mother – facing situations such as war, domestic violence, or mental health problems – may unwittingly pass her high levels of cortisol across the placenta to her fetus. There is some evidence that this can alter the fetal stress response. The infant can then be born with a more sensitive HPA stress response, which reacts more intensely to stress – social stress in particular – and is slower to recover from it. Over time, this over-reactive stress system may become an ongoing physiological condition, determining the individual's future vulnerability to stress and ways of coping with it.[30]

Once born, most babies continue to develop these important regulatory systems. Although functional at birth, the baby's HPA stress response is not normally very active in the early weeks of life. Although it is capable of kicking into action, mostly it remains 'hypoactive', relying on parents to manage threats. This provides a period of adjustment while the stress response 'thermostat' is getting 'set'. A baby in a safe and relaxed family is likely to set his or her stress response thermostat to react to stress at a different level from one who faces a threatening or anxiety-provoking environment, such as experiencing repeated separations from the primary attachment person in the first three months, or any kind of maltreatment by caregivers.[31]

In some situations, such as in a family where physical abuse has become the norm, or where a child in an institution is repeatedly ignored, the HPA system may eventually become 'blunted'. This means it becomes *less* rather than more reactive to stressful experiences (alongside diminished heart rate responses), as if these children's bodies had become disengaged from or even numb to adversity.[32] When this blunting is seen, the child's typical daily cortisol pattern is unusual: instead of the normal pattern of higher early morning cortisol, it is low at the start of the day. This state of chronic low cortisol has also been linked to increased inflammation.

These adaptations to a stressful situation at the start of life are not necessarily enduring; however, there is evidence that they do usually persist into adulthood. One study by Professor Marilyn Essex found that such epigenetic changes in babies due to early life stress were certainly detectable fifteen years later, when those infants had become teenagers.[33] Another American, endocrinologist Riya Kanherkar, summed up how such changes can affect cellular memory 'transiently, permanently or with a heritable alteration'.[34] In other words, epigenetic changes last for variable lengths of time, but once they have become established, there is a possibility that they will not only endure but also potentially be passed on to later generations and affect their future health.

Although we might think of these epigenetic changes as an attempt by the fetus to adapt to its immediate situation and biochemical signals from the mother, in the long run these early adjustments to parental stress can become counter-productive. As Fabiola Zucchi and her colleagues in a Canadian study put it, they 'may not support successful aging' because they can lead to an 'enhanced susceptibility to neurological and psychiatric disease'.[35]

The protective power of positive relationships

A small amount of stress during development can be helpful, positively increasing stress resistance later in life.[36] At least, this works for children who enjoy a reliable, soothing and comforting attachment relationship, which enables a child to recover rapidly from stressful experiences of various kinds. Notably, babies who enjoy the soothing qualities of breastfeeding for at least five months tend to become less reactive to stress than those who are not breastfed.[37] Even relatively strong threats to well-being, such as illness, a death in the family or a natural disaster, can often be tolerated when such experiences are buffered by warm and responsive parenting. However, if the baby is exposed to excessive or chronic stress in this early period, without adequately supportive parental care or where the adults themselves are the source of stress, as in abusive or neglectful relationships, this can become 'toxic stress' that undermines the effectiveness of the stress recovery system itself.[38]

In effect, other people are part of normal physiological

functioning, not only in infancy but even into adulthood. As the American neuroscientist Jay Schulkin explained, the healthy person is not defined by a particular level of the stress hormone cortisol but much more by his ability to use other people – in close relationships, or in social alliances – to comfort him, to reduce his stress and lower his cortisol level. This confident reliance on others is a sign of good regulation.[39] Or as psychologist Steve Porges and paediatric cardiologist Senta Furman put it, 'For humans, maturation does not lead to a total independence from others, but leads to ability to function independent of other people for short periods.'[40]

Although we develop more control over our bodies and our lives, we never achieve total independence. Even as adults, we go on needing friends and relatives to provide emotional support to restore our equilibrium when we are out of balance, and, equally, we depend on the wider social structures around us to meet basic needs, such as energy companies to provide warmth in our homes, supermarkets to organise the distribution of food, and the local council to remove or recycle our rubbish.

The effect of excessive stress on health

Crucially for our understanding of health, these early experiences of chronic or toxic stress can create a later vulnerability to disease. For example, early established hyper-responsiveness to stress increases both the likelihood of later anxiety and depression[41] and to a 'lifelong susceptibility to chronic disease', including metabolic (e.g. type 2 diabetes, obesity, neurological and cardiovascular disease).[42] It is also associated with turning off tumour suppressor genes, which may play a part in developing cancer.[43]

In recent decades, researchers have begun to investigate the mechanisms involved, and to establish just how a dysfunctional stress response might affect health. Two relatively new fields of research have begun to explore different ways in which early life stress can affect the developing immune system. One route is the impact of stress on our gut bacteria. Stress can reduce the diversity of these bacteria, which in turn can potentially affect their vital role in programming the early immune system. This will be explored further in Chapter Five.

Second, the immune system's inflammatory response – which can be triggered both by psychosocial stress as well as by the presence of pathogens[44] – can go into overdrive. Particularly in chronically unresolved stressful situations, the HPA stress response increasingly struggles to do its usual job. Instead of temporarily turning down the immune system's inflammatory response and then relying on negative feedback to bring it back into action when the stress is over, it seems to lose control of the inflammatory response. Certain immune cells, such as macrophages and T-cells, keep on producing the chemical messengers known as pro-inflammatory cytokines that stimulate further inflammation. This leaves the child with a double whammy: the body not only has an overactive HPA stress response, but also a chronically aggressive inflammatory response, which is increasingly thought to play a part in many disease processes.[45] Some have even calculated that stress and inflammation are common risk factors for as many as 75–90% of diseases.[46]

Self-control and health

The links between early psychological stress and long-term health were opened up by findings from the long-running Dunedin project. In 2004, the researchers decided to investigate the health of their original babies, who by now had turned into adults of thirty-two years of age. They found that 20% of the group had two or more of the physiological markers for ill health, such as high levels of a protein called CRP (c-reactive protein) that increases in response to inflammation, as well as a cluster of other health red flags, such as being overweight, having high blood pressure, high cholesterol and poor lung function.[47]

Looking back at the early data, the Dunedin researchers searched for links between these health-warning signs in adulthood and the individuals' early childhood histories. They were very surprised to discover the prime factor that linked early life with later health outcomes: the unhealthiest adults had been the children who, aged three and aged five, had demonstrated poor 'self-control' (a close relative of self-regulation) in their lab assessments. Even more surprising, a child's capacity for early self-control at the age of three was a better predictor of a whole range of future troubles than either socio-economic status or IQ. The Dunedin researchers, husband and wife team Avshalom Caspi and Terrie Moffitt, found it hard to believe. They admitted frankly that they did their 'best to pit self-control against *alternative* causes, but it survived all the tests we threw at it'.[48]

One explanation offered for the link between early self-control and later health was that, when restless, impulsive and inattentive children become teenagers, they are more likely to make poor choices, such as starting to smoke or take drugs, to have unprotected sex and risk pregnancy: in other words, they were less able to think ahead and take good care of their health. An alternative explanation might be that poor self-control could also be an indicator of how the pre-frontal cortex has developed in early life. 'Self-control' – as defined by Richie Poulton, another lynchpin of the Dunedin study – is about control of attention and of impulses, capacities that are strongly dependent on the early development of the pre-frontal cortex through attentive, firm and caring interactions in early life, as described by Allen Schore. Lack of self-control may, therefore, be the result of an unhappy early attachment relationship.

As well as affecting self-control, poor-quality early relationships are themselves stressful, and stress can affect the developing immune system, increasing the inflammatory response. Indeed, this was what Italian-born developmental psychobiologist and psychiatrist Andrea

Danese found when he explored the Dunedin data. He found that those children who in early life had been rejected by their parents, harshly disciplined, or sexually or physically abused, or had frequent changes of caregiver, had a significantly increased risk of 'clinically relevant' inflammatory CRP levels decades later, in adulthood.[49]

The ill health of our later years, which seems to many to be the result of the luck of the draw, may in reality have deep roots in our earliest experiences. As Terrie Moffitt summed it up, stressful early experiences 'might start a child on the long road to heart disease or dementia', with symptoms only emerging forty to seventy years later.[50]

Developmental origins of health and disease (DoHD)

The links between early development and later health are complex, as there are many sources of stress and many intertwined regulatory systems tangled in mutual feedback loops. However, the picture I have been trying to sketch would not be complete without including the role of nutrition and other breakthroughs in understanding that took place in the mid to late 1980s. Like the work to understand the developing stress response, this research focused on the impact of nutrition during pregnancy rather than psychological stress. In fact, poor nutrition is itself a form of stress for the organism trying to grow and survive.

The source of this breakthrough was the first British birth cohort study, called the Douglas study. Set up after the Second World War, it was a huge study of 17,415 babies born in the same week in 1946. Led by Dr James Douglas, its original remit had been to find out why the birth rate had been falling in the 1920s and 1930s, and whether the quality of maternity services played a part in this.

By the 1950s and 1960s, a new batch of researchers were interested in asking very different, more sociological, questions of the data. They went back to the original 'cohort' of people to explore links

Growing a person: a social, interactive view of health

between their early lives and later educational achievement and social mobility.

It was not until the 1980s, by which time the original 'Douglas babies' had become adults in their late thirties, that the relevance of the data to health became apparent.

Led by a sociologist called Michael Wadsworth, a new study set up in 1984 used the data to investigate links between the recorded health of adults and their health as babies. Wadsworth found a startling correlation between adult blood pressure and a person's weight at birth: the smaller the baby, the higher his or her adult blood pressure. To him, this novel finding suggested that poor nutrition (and/or smoking) as far back as pregnancy might be affecting health many years later. This was a challenge to the belief that current 'lifestyle choices' are the main cause of disease.

Coincidentally, a doctor and epidemiologist called David Barker had been doing an entirely independent study at the same time, which reached identical conclusions. While a professor at the University of Southampton, Barker had worked hard to locate and gain access to a batch of health records of children born in Hertfordshire between 1911 and 1930. After studying the details of their early infancy from these records, he investigated what had happened to the men in old age, sixty or seventy years later. He found out who had already died and their causes of death, and traced the survivors. He too found that the adults most likely to have higher blood pressure and to be at greatest risk of heart disease in older age had been born at a low birthweight. As Barker put it, those who had poor-quality early nutrition, both in utero and in early life, had less robust hearts – they were 'built on the cheap'.

Just as Charles Darwin and Alfred Russel Wallace reached similar conclusions about natural selection at the same time in the 1840s, one had to publish first. In this case it was Wadsworth. David Barker immediately contacted Wadsworth and is reported to have said 'You scooped me'.[51] However, David Barker went on to become the better-known individual and a tireless promotor

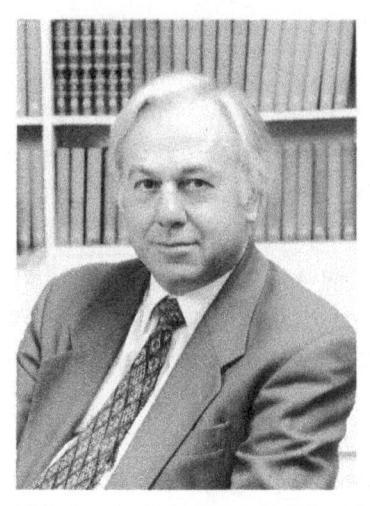

Professor David Barker, British pioneer of the 'developmental origins of health and disease' (DoHD) hypothesis

of the 'developmental origins of health and disease' (DoHD) hypothesis.

Described as a warm, humorous man whose department 'was alive with banter and fun', Barker was passionate about the possibility his research had opened up, that disease might be prevented. He explained his outlook in an analogy about cars:

> Across the world there is now general agreement that human beings are like motor cars. They break down either because they are being driven on rough roads or because they were badly made in the first place.
>
> Rolls-Royce cars do not break down no matter where they are being driven. How do we build stronger people? By improving the nutrition of babies in the womb. The greatest gift we could give the next generation is to improve the nutrition and growth of girls and young women.[52]

In particular, the way that girls and women are physically nourished, and the nourishment they then provide for their babies, is turning out to be a central concern for future health. While hearts may be 'built on the cheap', so too can many other organs, such as the pancreas, kidneys, and ovaries. When they lack good nutritional support for their growth in the womb, they can end up smaller. This means they may not last as well and are more susceptible to diseases, such as diabetes or cardiovascular disease, in an individual's later years, when ageing begins to undermine their efficiency.

A century of learning

In the century since the 1920s 'Decade of the Child' much has been discovered. A new developmental paradigm has established that human psychological development is highly interactive; more recently, that human health is also fundamentally affected by the emotional stresses of human interaction as well as by stresses such as poor nutrition.

By spelling out just how a new human being is grown, the developmental approach makes us more aware of what can go wrong, starting from conception, or even earlier due to the epigenetic transmission of negative environmental effects (such as bad diet, stress or pollution) via sperm and egg cells.

'Growing' humans might seem an odd way to describe it, as if we were plants or trees. However, just as any gardener knows that plant health depends on the quality of the soil, human development and health also depends on the quality of the environment, particularly the early environment. And for highly social animals like humans, the 'soil' in which we grow is not only physical but also a matrix of social and emotional resources.

Regrettably, despite a wealth of research, the medical profession has been slow to adapt to this knowledge. Medical students still to this day learn little in their training about the importance of early nutrition or the impact of early stress and trauma on lifelong health; such research is not part of the key curriculum. How many of us even know what our birth weight was, let alone are using it as a way to gauge whether we should be regularly checking our blood pressure?

Yet these aspects of the developmental process are crucial to understanding both ill health and how to prevent it. Our bodies and our biology, as well as our selves, are responsive to our environments – the food we eat, the relationships we experience, and the cultural and political environment in which we are immersed. These processes are constantly changing as we change and are changed. Turning to look at this process of development in detail – what does it mean to say that the body is constructed in a relational and interactive way?

PART TWO

The Body Under Construction

3.
Starting with cells

> *'Consider, for example, the distinction between a living cell and a dead cell: at a single instant, a living cell and a dead cell may contain precisely the same catalogue of component molecules in the same concentrations; the parts catalogue is the same for both the living and the dead. It is not the parts themselves, but the dynamics of their interactions that distinguish the living from the dead. The living cell goes on interacting as a reactive system and the dead cell decays into disintegration.'*
>
> I. Cohen and D. Harel, *Journal of the Royal Society*

A human being starts with a cell – or even earlier, with the process of interaction between sperm and egg. The spur to growth and development is the spark as two things come together and coordinate with each other, whether that is at the level of cells, individuals, or groups. Positive interaction enables new things to happen. A supportive environment provides the energy needed for growth.

The very definition of a living system, as opposed, say, to a rock, is that it has an interactive relationship with its environment. Life does not consist of an abstract piece of DNA or a cell or a person in splendid isolation; its aliveness comes from being part of a 'metabolic network'. In other words, a cell exists only by being part of an environment that supplies the energy and resources to develop. The quality of that environment matters. Although plants can grow on stony ground, they tend to be straggling weeds. In a similar vein,

1,001 Days

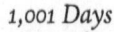

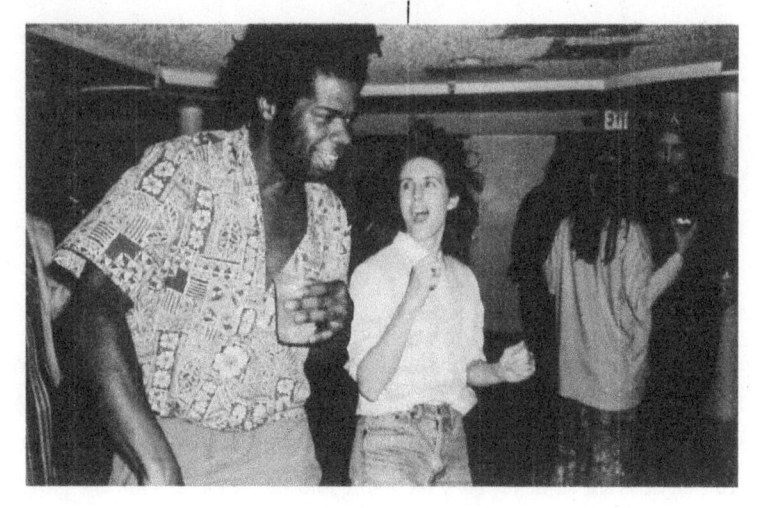

The joy of interacting

people born into hostile circumstances can survive, but their life is less likely to flourish and last a long time.

Every cell needs energy to stay alive by taking in elements of the environment, processing them and expelling the waste products. Cells have boundaries called membranes, which are loose and porous, peppered with 'innumerable channels, gates and pores' that are designed to let in oxygen, nutrients and certain proteins, while limiting access to other substances, such as ions, sugars and amino acids. All life forms – from bacteria to humans – are 'open systems', dependent on the environment that surrounds them.*[1]

As complex multicellular creatures, humans are interactive at many levels. When we are born, many systems start to become operational as they interact with the outside world. We survive by breathing air, we generate energy by digesting food, we depend on the parents who nurture us, and on the society which organises our world. And, in turn, our breathing releases carbon dioxide back into the environment, we generate heat through our movement, and we

---

* Viruses are a different matter, as they are pieces of DNA which survive as parasites on a living cell – no one seems quite sure if they count as 'alive' or not.

alter other people through our interactions with them. There is a constant movement of taking things in, processing them, and sending the waste out.

Surprisingly, bacteria cells also communicate with each other and co-ordinate their behaviour via chemical signals and even, it has recently been discovered, signal to one another electrically – using electrically charged particles to organise and synchronise activities across large expanses, albeit at a tortoise-like pace compared to human neurons. They also gather together in communities, building 'sticky organic superstructures around themselves' called biofilm.[2]

Interaction makes things happen. Human sexual interaction connects two bodies to potentially make a third, body to body, which is normally an act of mutual agency fuelled by the energy of desire for pleasure and connection. From that encounter, there is the possibility of new life. However, there is a randomness about it as nature casually overproduces sperm and expects many to die en route: thousands of sperm set off in search of a receptive egg, but only one will succeed, if that. The more sperm a man produces and the more mobile they are, the better the chances that one will reach the egg and fertilise it successfully.

Nature generates a profusion of possibilities – many sperm, many seedlings, many neurons, many people. This provides more chances that there will be some whose characteristics suit the environment of the day or who can successfully adapt, and will survive.

Evolution

Those who survive are not 'fit' in any absolute sense of being 'the best', but only the best suited to survive in their current environment. For example, in 1848, relatively early in the English industrial revolution, most English peppered moths were a light colour. Less

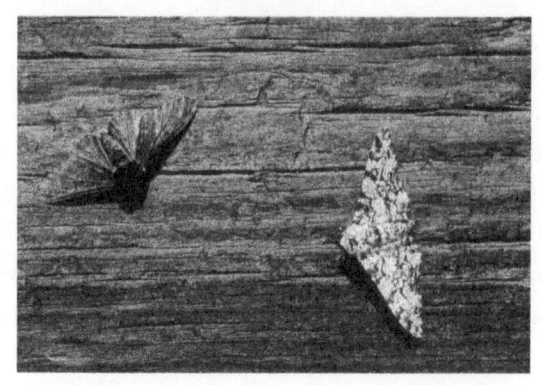

Contrasting dark and light peppered moths

than 2% had a dark colour. But as industrialisation spread, the landscape changed, and soot from the factories darkened the pale birch trees where the pale moths lived. It became more dangerous to be a light-coloured moth; the pale colour stood out against the dark sooty trees and light moths could be picked off more easily by the birds, who ate more of them.

By 1898, the vast majority of moths in Manchester and other industrial cities had become dark moths. The dark moths were the ones who had survived and reproduced; the other moths died out.

For people living in the nineteenth century, the Darwinian idea of evolution was a major challenge to the dominant belief of the day that there was a natural hierarchy of life forms created by God, with humans at the pinnacle. It was hard for many to accept that humans were only one kind of animal among many. Few people, including Darwin himself, wanted to take his ideas on board. One apocryphal story relates that a bishop's wife, when told about Darwin's theory, declared: 'Let's hope it's not true; but if it is true, let's hope it does not become widely known'.[3]

More recent work in evolutionary psychology has explored how our own human bodies have adapted over the centuries. The unique human brain, in particular, is probably the result of adapting to life in ever more complex social groups. Some particularly fascinating work has been done by the neuroscientist Jaak Panksepp, looking at the emotional systems of the brain. I heard Jaak Panksepp speak in London in 2000, when his work in 'affective neuroscience' was novel and pioneering. He was an impressively sincere and quietly spoken man from a rural background in north-eastern Europe. He became a child refugee in the 1940s (when the Soviets invaded his home country), and settled in the USA. By the 1990s, he had become a scientist, in the forefront of using new technology to understand how emotions worked – a field that had previously been neglected.

Panksepp identified what he thought was the most ancient and primal emotion system in the brain, calling it the SEEKING system. He identified areas in the brain, including the nucleus accumbens (which releases the neurotransmitter dopamine involved in seeking rewards of various kinds), together with other linked structures, such as the hypothalamus (involved in many functions such as appetite, sleep and regulating hormones), as the network which is responsible for our basic drive – the energy to move forward, to approach, our motivation to survive and to procreate.[4]

Panksepp speculated that, over time, this basic drive got elaborated into more specialised emotion networks. As his colleague Doug Watt explains, this is how evolution works: it builds on what is already there. It 'tweaks and enhances the existing operations a bit here and there to manage the new adaptive context'.[5] It is likely that, as mammals became more social, they increasingly found it useful to build extensions to their SEEKING system, a bit like you would build an extension to your house when you need more room. These brain extensions provided shortcuts to the most frequently experienced social emotions. They set up 'core routines' to trigger key emotion networks, such as for anger (including aggression), fear (including anxiety and the pain of separation) and for nurturing impulses (including both maternal and sexual love bonds, as well as the joy of playfulness). These networks were then at the ready to organise appropriate behaviour more quickly and effectively.

From an evolutionary point of view, our much prized 'higher' cognitive activity is a further refinement of these emotional routines. It has evolved as a response to a changing way of living. While much of life is lived in a non-conscious way – our bodies do the work of digesting food, circulating blood, sleeping, excreting, breathing, and feeling emotions without needing to be conscious – we do need to make more choices when the social world gets more complex, and it becomes more difficult to manage the stresses and strains of living among other human beings.[6] In response to this more complicated social world, connections in the areas of the brain most used for social behaviour are strengthened and consolidated. This expanded connectivity enabled people to anticipate and predict what other people might do, and work out how to co-operate with each other. The more effectively they could do this, the more intelligently they could behave.

New growth

However, all this complexity is built up from tiny beginnings. The story of each human life begins with a sperm cell and egg cell connecting to form a single cell.

When this cell finds a sustaining environment in the mother's body, it embeds itself in the wall of her womb. Then, like a manic knitter, it begins its long, repetitive chore of endlessly dividing and multiplying to make new cells. After about five days, there are enough cells to form a blastocyst, which, like a squatter, gets its energy supplies from the free nutrients (glucose, hormones and oxygen) floating in its mother's reproductive tract. However, there is still only a 50/50 chance it will go on to become an embryo. Around half the blastocysts won't make it, often because they are defective in some way.

The successful blastocyst multiplies cells rapidly. By five weeks after fertilisation, the single cell has grown into a cluster of about 500 cells. Now it is sufficiently organised to plan for survival. Its first task is to set up a system that can generate enough energy to enable more complex growth. It does this by dividing into a placenta and an embryo. The placenta becomes the storage and exchange unit, available to the embryo as a safe source of fluids from the mother's bloodstream – her carbon dioxide, proteins, lipids, hormones, antibodies, viruses – and a place where toxins, such as the mother's stress hormones, are normally filtered out. Using this source of energy, cells can go on multiplying, to the point where there is enough tissue to start forming a body.

Yet rapid growth is one aspect of the whole picture. The process of building a body (and a self) also depends on selection: from abundant possibilities, choices are necessary; some potentials have to be repressed, blocked, or discarded. Just as in creating a sculpture (or in writing a book), the shape emerges as much from what is eliminated, and from the spaces between things. In growing tissue, these spaces also have as much of a role to play as the tissue itself. For example, early in development, the fetus has only a flipper shape at the end of its arms. Around eight weeks' gestation, this is sculpted into a hand with fingers. This is achieved by cells in the finger area inducing the cell death (apoptosis) of the cells in between the fingers, enabling flipper-like hands to develop distinct fingers.

Stem cells

As the mass of cells grow, they need to get organised into particular forms and functions; they cannot just grow. The earliest cells – the stem cells – are ready to be drafted in to build a bigger, more complex unit, by specialising and becoming any part of the body that is needed, e.g. a skin cell, a lung cell, or a retinal cell.

How do these first cells decide which type of cell they will become? This is a complex process. Stem cells can be drafted by the collective to become different kinds of cells depending on where they find themselves in the whole, i.e. their relationship to each other. For example, if they find themselves located on the outside of a bunch of cells, they may turn into skin cells; if they are located in the brain, they become nerve cells or neurons. There is a sort of 'peer pressure' to develop in particular ways: 'the cells at the front end of the neural plate induce the cells further forward to form a nose and then the cells on the side to form eyes'. Each cell's fate is decided collectively: 'how cells specialise mostly depends on their neighbours, chemical signals from the rest of the organism or environmental factors'. One population of cells interacts with another population and alters each other.[7]

Cells pull and push each other, responding either to other nearby cells or to stimulation or provocation from the wider environment. As the developmental biologist Lewis Wolpert put it, 'Cells need to know both what their neighbours have to say, and must also listen to long-range chemical signals like hormones that might be sent out from distant sources'.[8] They emit chemical signals and receive them from other cells, picking up on small changes in the intensity of the signal, and in the concentration of chemicals being emitted.

When cells receive a signal, they respond by triggering the release of proteins called 'transcription factors'. These 'master regulators' choose which parts of the DNA script it will be useful to activate, and which to turn off. They encourage production of some proteins and not others, guiding the stem cells to become particular kinds of cells. However, the genetic coding that sets a developmental process in motion need not specify its final structure – 'only enough to move the process along to a point where a fresh element (such as a hormone or a neurotransmitter newly accessible to the developing structure) can provide further specifications'.[9]

Different types of cell

Cells also have built-in self-maintenance. They respond to everyday wear and tear by renewing themselves. Some cells, such as skin cells, blood cells or cells that line the gut, need to be renewed on a regular basis. For this purpose, the organism stores virgin stem cells in store cupboards or 'niches' all over the body, so that they can make new cells to replace cells that have become damaged or died. The stem cell divides, keeping one 'daughter' stem cell in storage, while the other gets drafted in to making the repair.

Other cells, such as fat cells, kidney cells or muscle cells, are more fixed in number and do not get renewed after a baby is born (though muscle cells will need a constant turnover of protein every day to maintain their function). Most brain neurons are more or less fixed in number too, apart from a few exceptions. The majority of brain cells need to stay as they are, in order to preserve their knowledge, which is held in stable neural networks.

However, the energy needed for cell division and replenishment begins to fade with time. While the body systems are buzzing with energy and optimum functioning in the years leading up to reproduction, they become less efficient the more often they divide. As Harvard Medical School professor Anthony Komaroff sums it up: 'Each time a cell divides, a little bit of the telomere – DNA at the tip of each chromosome – is lost. Thus, telomeres of young cells are longer than the telomeres of middle-aged cells, which in turn are longer than the telomeres of old cells. When the telomeres become very short, the cell can no longer divide, and it dies.'[10] Muscles waste, the brain functions less well, eyes get cloudy, plaques form in blood vessels. Ageing happens so that the human stock can be renewed and new adaptations can take place to the environment. It, too, is an evolutionary strategy.

The collective decides

The cooperation at the heart of development can seem a bit alien to our individualistic understanding of ourselves. It is an extraordinary phenomenon, a collective endeavour organising around 37 trillion cells to form the many different tissues and organs that are needed. All cells serve the needs of the organism as a whole in different ways, but there is no individual 'director' of this process. Billions of cells are brought together to make tissues, then tissues are pulled together to make organs, and in turn organs are connected to make systems.[11] For example, the digestive system is a process where a range of organs and structures – oesophagus, stomach, intestines – cooperate to achieve the objective of digesting food.

Furthermore, these multicellular organisms elaborated existing 'whole body systems' of cells into the endocrine, immune, circulating and nervous systems, to ensure that these living entities could collaborate to meet challenges and survive. As the renowned Portuguese neuroscientist and prize-winning author Antonio Damasio put it, 'without the whole body systems the complex structures and functions of multicellular organisms would not be viable'. In his view, 'The body . . . is part of a massively complex organism made up of cooperative systems, which are made up of cooperative organs, which are made up of cooperative cells, which are made up of cooperative molecules, which are made up of cooperative atoms built from cooperative particles'.[12] As he commented in an earlier book, 'If this sounds familiar and makes you think of human societies, it is because it should. The resemblances are staggering.'[13]

The stem cell expert Neil Theise explores the analogy further: 'cells give rise to the emergent phenomena of living, moving people. But people, in turn, interact and give rise emergently to the organisation of social structures such as cities, cultures and civilisations.'[14] This, too, involves constant negotiation and re-positioning as individuals and groupings shape and limit us. We cannot live outside these social structures, which implicitly organise what we can do and be. For example, as psychologist Vivien Burr elaborates, 'in a capitalist society competition is fundamental; society is structured around individuals and organisations that compete with each other for jobs, markets, etc.'. She continues: 'where competition is a fundamental feature of social and economic life, what you will get is competitive people'.[15] Just as the cell responds to its position in the body, so does each individual's response to his or her social environment determine what he or she will become. Human social selves acquire an identity as individuals in a similarly collective way – each 'self' is defined in response to the people nearby. Through their mirroring and communicating and interacting, some potential qualities within the individual's DNA are evoked and developed, while others do not emerge. This developmental model is different from the idea of genes dictating what we become.

For the cognitive scientist Daniel Dennett, the rapid division and multiplication of cells appears alien without a directing self: 'An impersonal, unreflective, robotic, mindless little scrap of molecular machinery is the ultimate basis of all the agency, and hence meaning, and hence consciousness, in the universe.' As he puts it, 'All that hustle and bustle, and yet there's nobody home . . .'[16] Certainly *individual* agency is not in evidence, at the level of the single cell, but in more complex plant and animal life, the organism is multicellular, part of a multicellular community with a collective mind of some sort.

An alternative way of looking at it is to recognise that the individual organism is ultimately directed by its environment and its relationship to its environment. It is part of a bigger whole. While individual organisms are distinctive, because they each have a unique genome and a unique history, their uniqueness is paradoxically largely determined by their response to the environment around them. The driving force is the whole environment, not the individual part.

And in the first nine months of development (and beyond), that environment is the mother's body. How then does the human mother, and her own environment, shape the development of her fetus?

4.
Growing inside mother's body

> *'Vague as fog and looked for like mail.*
> *Farther off than Australia.*
> *Bent-backed Atlas, our travelled prawn.*
> *Snug as a bud and at home*
> *Like a sprat in a pickle jug.'*
>
> Sylvia Plath, 'You're'

Mother and fetus affect each other

The interactive principle of development is operating from the start between the fetus and its mother. Just as cells communicate and organise themselves in relation to each other, so does biochemical communication between mother and fetus shape the way we develop in the womb. Although these processes are off the radar, outside awareness, they are already creating the unique story of each new individual and influencing his or her future life.

From the start of a pregnancy, the embryo – then fetus – is interacting not only with the mother's body, and its state of health, but also indirectly with her social world. Even such mundane aspects of her reality, such as the availability of fresh vegetables in her neighbourhood, how much traffic and noise surrounds her, whether she has friends or family nearby, and whether her employer expects her to work long hours, can potentially alter the experience of her fetus in the womb. As the pregnancy progresses, each fetus responds to biochemical cues from its mother's body that tell it how much energy from food is likely to be available, as well as likely levels of stress in the life ahead. If she is relaxed, well-fed and well-supported, the fetus will be 'programmed' for a relatively low stress, high nutrition life. But if she is highly stressed, over-eats, under-eats, smokes, drinks, takes drugs, or is ill, her fetus will do its best to adapt to this negative information from the mother in order to survive.

The relationship between mother and fetus is a two-way process. The mother also has to adapt to the fetus. From the start of pregnancy, the fetus is making its own silent demands on the mother's body. In response, her body systems rev up: her blood plasma volume expands, blood glucose adjusts, her cardiac output increases, her cholesterol and lipid levels rise, along with increased appetite hormone (leptin) and greater consumption of oxygen, as she responds to the needs of the new organism that is part of her yet distinct from her.[1] While unlikely to be aware of these changes, she may be aware of her changing body through the side effects of increased hormones. Many women experience the effects of oestrogen and progesterone as strange tastes in the mouth, nausea and tiredness, or are aware of their growing breasts. She may also have new anxieties about the future changes in her life that this baby will bring, such as financial worries, the need to return to work, concerns about the impact on her relationship with her partner or how she will manage caring for a baby.

Mother and fetus manage resources through the placenta

Growing a new life uses energy. The first source of energy, as outlined in the previous chapter, is generated by the cell burrowing into the wall of the womb to get nutrients directly from the stored sugar (glycogens) and glycoproteins secreted by the lining of the womb.

Growing inside mother's body

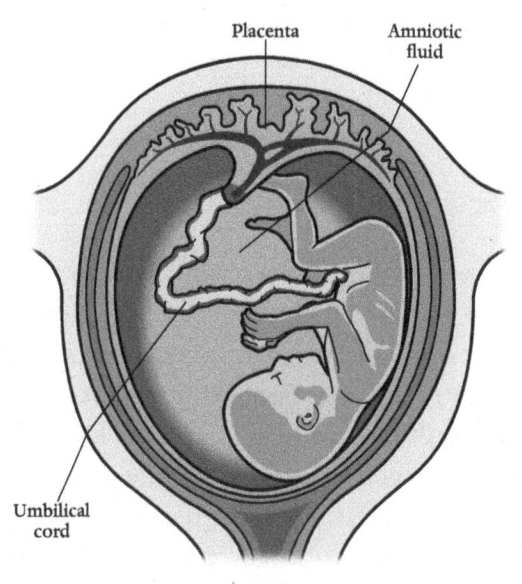

A fetus growing in the womb, attached to the placenta

These supply enough energy to support the earliest development of the very first weeks of a pregnancy.

Soon, however, the growing embryo needs more. So between around eight to eleven weeks, the mother and embryo jointly construct a bigger, more ambitious structure, called the placenta, that will take over the delivery of energy and other nutrients in the mother's arterial blood.

The placenta is a flat, thick pancake full of blood; it looks like a slab of liver.* Operating as a sort of halfway house between mother and fetus – it is attached both to the lining of the mother's womb and also connected to the fetus via the umbilical cord – without the two making direct contact.

This allows the fetus to have access to the good things in the mother's blood while also screening out potentially harmful substances in her blood, such as bacterial infections, drugs or stress hormones. However, if levels of pathogens are too high, the

---

* Some enthusiasts even choose to cook and eat it after the birth.

placenta's ability to manage them can be overwhelmed and these substances can cross the placenta and reach the fetus.

Building a body

When the mother is healthy, the placenta acts as a remarkable food store, which has everything the fetus needs to develop. A well-nourished mother usually doesn't have to do or eat anything different for the placenta to effortlessly share her own body's nutrients with her fetus. As long as she eats enough nourishing food – sufficient protein, leafy greens and pulses that supply folate – as well as food that supplies vitamins, such as B2 (found in green vegetables and dairy) or B3 (found in fish, chicken, nuts, whole grains), the new organism can grow and flourish. Via the umbilical cord, the fetus will draw on its mother's blood to access everything it needs, such as essential supplies of oxygen, cholesterol, protein and fatty acids, as well as important micronutrients, such as folic acid, iron, choline and iodine.

Cholesterol might seem a surprising essential ingredient, since it has been demonised in recent years due to its association with heart disease. However, our livers (and gut) make cholesterol for good reason. It is a versatile substance that contributes to the production of highly important vitamin D, as well as cortisol and bile acids. In fact, it is an integral component of every cell in our bodies. In the first few months of pregnancy, the fetus draws on a placental supply of waxy, fatty yellow cholesterol to build firm cell walls.

First things first

One of the first tasks of the developing organism is to form the vascular system and the heart – the starter motor that will pump blood around the organism so that these nutrients can reach all its parts. Incredibly, it starts beating as early as three weeks after conception (known as gestational week five of the pregnancy, around the time when the woman's period is first missed), although it may not be functional till around week sixteen.[2] Despite being as tiny as a poppy seed, it already starts contracting, sending blood around the tiny embryo. Watching a video of this speck of tissue starting to pulsate and become animated feels like watching life begin.

In the early weeks of pregnancy, many structures start off as a tube that gradually takes more precise form. This is true of the digestive system, which can be described as a tube that stretches from mouth to anus, as well as the neural tube that will become a brain and spinal cord. Other structures are more like small buds that grow into distinct organs, such as the liver, kidneys, pancreas and stomach. Each has its own slightly different developmental timetable.

Some organs develop more slowly than others. The brain, in particular, takes longer to form its structures. The stem cells that form the human brain have the enormous task of generating 86 billion permanent neurons. Most of them are formed by mid gestation. By the end of the second trimester, the lowest part of the brain, the brainstem that manages breathing, heart rate and blood pressure, is maturing, as well as structures like the hypothalamus (which controls the autonomic nervous system which regulates temperature, appetite and so on) and amygdala (involved in emotional reactivity).

Getting ready to launch

The last few weeks of pregnancy are a period of intense preparation for life outside the womb. As the dramatic moment approaches when the baby will be born into a world requiring the breathing of oxygen, the fetal lungs start to mature (from around the twenty-sixth week to thirty-sixth week). In these later stages of pregnancy, the baby's brain also starts to get organised to deal with the prospect of a massive influx of new sensory and social information after birth. Neurons now begin an intense process of connecting with each other via 'synapses' that can pass electrical or chemical signals between themselves to convey information.

To assist this process, the mother's body once again generates extra cholesterol to make myelin, another vital fatty substance, that helps the fetal nervous system to work efficiently. Myelin is often compared to the insulation on electric wiring, as it gets wrapped around the signalling end (axons) of the brain cells, speeding up the electrical and biochemical signalling between neurons.*

In the last few weeks of pregnancy (by about gestational week thirty-four), almost 40,000 new brain synapses are formed every second, connecting up the brain's neurons.[3] Nor is this the end of the story, as further rapid synaptic connection will also occur in the early months and years after birth, then continue at a slower pace into adolescence and beyond.

Other changes are also taking place in the mother's body to prepare for the needs of the baby who will soon be born. Towards the end of pregnancy, the mother's gut and vaginal bacteria become less diverse, while, at the same time, her level of bifidobacteria increases; this is the gut bacteria that the newborn baby will shortly need to process the special sugars in breast milk, which will potentially be the next source of energy for growth.[4]

---

* Despite these useful functions, it seems to be important for the mother's cholesterol levels to stay within a balanced range: there is some evidence that when mothers have a very low, or a very high, level of cholesterol, there is an increased risk of premature birth. This matters as prematurity is the single largest cause of death in the first month of life. However, a prospective study of pregnant Ghanaian women by Brietta Oaks and her colleagues narrowed down such findings, discovering that riskier, shorter pregnancies were linked only to low levels of 'good cholesterol' (HDL (high-density lipoprotein)), not to low total cholesterol. Hopefully, further research will clarify the meaning of these results in future.

Also in later pregnancy, heightened levels of the female hormone oestrogen, generated by the placenta, trigger other changes in the mother's body. Some fascinating work done by Dutch neuroscientist Elseline Hoekzema has demonstrated that this increased oestrogen correlates with a remodelling of the brain's neural networks, as the woman reshapes her sense of herself to become a mother. Hoekzema found that at this time the brain loses grey matter volume in certain areas in order to streamline their operations and to become more efficient at the tasks that matter most. In late pregnancy, this 'pruning' occurs in areas of the brain called the default mode network and ventral striatum, which are central to emotional processing. This enables mothers to focus on their fetus as a separate person with its own emotional needs.

It also rewards mothers with a rush of extra feel-good dopamine that can help generate positive maternal feelings and can strengthen the bond with her baby– a phenomenon that lasts for at least the next two years. Touchingly, Hoekzema herself became a mother twice over during the years of conducting this research.[5]

Towards the end of pregnancy, increased oestrogen also helps to prepare for the birth and beyond. It helps her uterus to make the contractions that will push the baby out at birth and also prepares the mother's breasts for breastfeeding. Also in the last three months of pregnancy, the placenta passes on the mother's

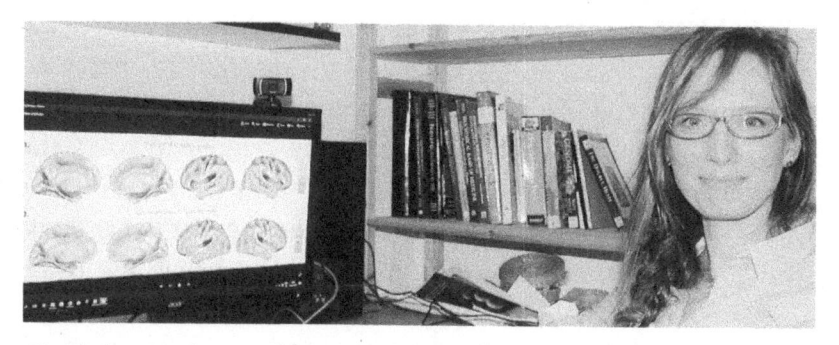

Dr Elseline Hoekzema, the Dutch neuroscientist who identified the impact of pregnancy on a mother's brain

antibodies to the fetus, which will provide it with some temporary protection from the dangerous bacteria and viruses soon to be encountered in the world, before the baby's own immune system starts to develop.

Healthy mother, healthy placenta

However, not all placentas are the same. Each new mother's body brings its own life story, starting with influences on her own development when she was a fetus, her own birthweight, as well as her current height, weight and health – all of which can have an impact on the health of her placenta and on the fetus that relies on it for sustenance.

A healthy placenta protects the fetus. On the other hand, a placenta may not function as well if the mother's health is compromised in some way. Health issues that can potentially undermine the best functioning of the placenta include smoking, maternal infection, high blood pressure or living with a great deal of stress. In particular, being significantly over- or underweight brings increased risk. This is usually defined as having a Body Mass Index (BMI) of over 25 or under 18. While being extremely underweight is relatively rare, these days being overweight is not rare at all – it is an extraordinary fact that most adult women in the UK and USA are now overweight or obese.* In the worst case scenario, the placenta may end up showing signs of increased inflammation and oxidative stress, becoming prematurely calcified, small or enlarged. Then the fetus may struggle to access the supplies it needs to grow and develop well.[6] For example, a mother who is obese may be less able to transfer iron supplies to her fetus, with some evidence suggesting iron-deficient babies are more

---

* In the UK, 63% of adults were overweight or obese in 2021 and the figures are even higher in the USA.

irritable and harder to soothe as newborns, slower to process information, have slower motor coordination and are more socially inhibited and wary.[7]

The size of placenta is correlated with the birth weight of the baby: small placenta, small baby. The exception to that rule is that, in some situations of poor nutrition, the placenta may instead grow larger than usual as it struggles to extract whatever nutrients it can. Both small and large placentas are linked to chronic disease. As with the story of Goldilocks and the three bears, placental growth needs to be 'just right': not too big, not too small.

Growing organs

The unhealthy diet that is currently the norm in richer countries – dominated by red meat, sugar and processed food instead of fresh fruit, vegetables, pulses, whole grains, nuts and fish – affects our well-being as adults, but can have a potentially huge impact on a developing fetus. When the mother is not getting enough to eat, or is eating food lacking in nutrition – particularly in the early months of pregnancy – the organs that are developing in this period may not grow well.[8] For example, a lack of leafy greens in the diet, leading to a lack of folate, has been associated with impaired fetal growth and, in some cases, pre-term delivery. In fact, folate is so vital it has now become a recommended supplement for all pregnant mothers.

In particular, cardiovascular disease has been linked back to an inadequate diet at an early stage of pregnancy. A lack of nutrition can lead to growing a smaller heart with fewer heart muscle cells (cardiomyocytes), which, it has been speculated, 'may lead to compromised cardiac function later in life'.[9] Certainly the evidence of the Dutch Hunger Winter of 1944–5 seemed to corroborate this theory. During this period of German occupation, the Dutch were starving from lack of food and could access only around 400–800

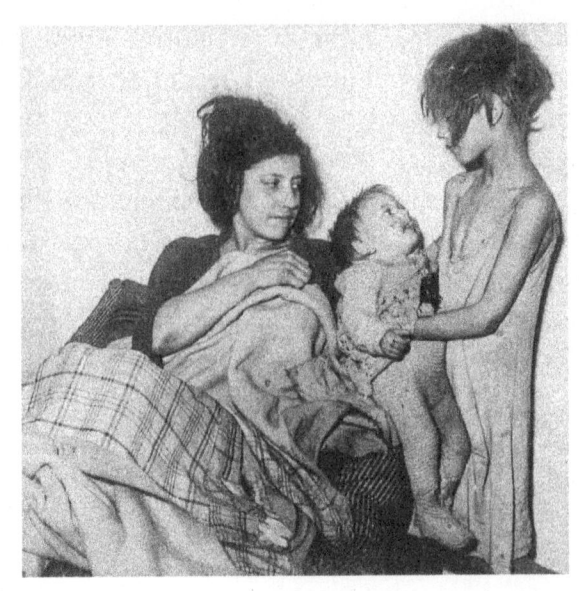

A family suffering during the Dutch Hunger Winter of 1944–5

calories a day. Starving mothers who were then in early pregnancy had babies who, as adults, had higher rates of cardiovascular disease.[10] This did not apply to the offspring of mothers who were at a later stage of pregnancy during the famine, showing how significant developmental timing is.

Diets seriously lacking in nutrition in early pregnancy have also been linked to heart defects, although these conditions are rare (about 1% of births) and can have other causes, such as a rubella infection (one infection that does cross the placenta), exposure to alcohol, nicotine, or medical drugs – or just genetic bad luck.[11] Whatever the cause or complex mix of factors involved, these conditions are devastating for their families, who are unlikely to be aware of the long-term consequences of inadequate nutrition in the first few weeks of pregnancy, especially as researchers, clinicians and policy experts themselves have given this 'too little attention', according to one eminent group of fifteen US medical professionals.[12]

One reason for this neglect of nutrition is that, for at least the last twenty years or so, since the sequencing of the human genome, research has largely been focused on understanding genetic causes for congenital heart disease (CHD), the most common birth defect. As Jacinta Kalisch-Smith and her colleagues at Oxford University argue, 'despite these efforts and the discovery of almost 100 genes associated with human CHD, routine whole-genome sequencing of large numbers of CHD patients and their families has only provided genetic explanations for around 30% of CHD cases ... Thus, scientific interest has returned to non-genetic cases and uncovering the environmental causes of CHD'.[13] This is a cause for optimism, as one major 'environmental' cause of heart disease is the quality of our diet. Having an awareness of a possible predisposition to heart disease in later life might give those affected a renewed energy and determination in making changes to their diets. However difficult it might be to turn our dietary habits around, improving them for preconception and pregnant women in particular is an objective that should be achievable.

The heart is not the only organ that can be affected by inadequate nutrition in pregnancy. For example, a lack of protein (or of particular 'micronutrients', such as zinc, vitamin A or iron) in the mother's diet can affect the developing kidneys, leading to fewer 'nephrons' – kidney tissues that filter out waste products from the blood and keep it in good condition. Since nephron number is already established at birth and doesn't increase after that (unless the baby is born premature), this can open up potential risk for hypertension, kidney disease or renal dysfunction in adulthood.[14] There is also evidence that stress or poor nutrition that leads to serious growth restriction may also result in a loss of cells in the fetal pancreas, or to smaller pancreatic 'islets', an area of the pancreas where insulin is made. Insulin plays a vital role in managing blood sugar levels and letting sugar into cells to generate energy.[15] If the process does not work well, it can result in diabetes and high blood sugar that can damage blood vessels and nerves.

Inadequate nutrition tends to have its most powerful impact on organs when they are at a formative stage of development. Certain adult health conditions can be traced back to this early 'programming', as it is called. David Barker, who we met in an earlier chapter, first established this in the 1980s in his research on groups of British children born in the 1920s and 1930s. It revealed strong links between an increased risk of cardiovascular disease, high blood pressure, stroke, osteoporosis, diabetes and metabolic disorders in adulthood and a low birth weight.[16]

In the early years of the 'Barker hypothesis', there was considerable resistance to Barker's discoveries. His story of the fetal origins of adult disease seemed to challenge the accepted view that either genes or current adult diet and lifestyle were the principal causes of ill health. However, Barker doggedly pursued his hypothesis and built a research unit at Southampton University with links around the world. Over subsequent decades, they (and others) have constructed a fuller picture, including an understanding of how post-natal experiences might add to disease risk. They highlighted the way that a poorly nourished fetus could develop a 'thrifty phenotype', adapting to the scarcity of nutrition by learning to store precious surplus calories as invisible fat around the abdominal organs (visceral fat), much like a human version of the camel's hump. In some circumstances, this may be a useful adaptation to an impoverished food environment in the womb, preparation for a future environment where food is scarce. However, it could become a health liability when the 'thrifty' baby is then exposed to a post-natal environment it was not expecting, awash with high calorie food, and then rapidly lays down large amounts of fat rather than muscle mass. In this scenario, it is the mis-match between the expectations of an underfed fetus and a plentiful early childhood food environment that leads to weight problems.

The wrong food and obesity

Obesity has become an increasing problem since Barker's pioneering work of the 1980s. The food environment has changed dramatically, bringing new health dangers for fetuses and children. A new form of malnutrition has emerged – not based on a lack of food but on over-supply of high calorie, nutritionally empty food. This is spreading across the globe, even reaching remote places such as the Kathmandu Valley in Nepal, where babies and toddlers are now getting a quarter of their calories from junk food, such as instant noodles, sugary drinks and crisps.[17] Some pundits predict that a majority of today's children will be obese by the time they are thirty-five years old,[18] negatively affecting many of their body systems and increasing their risk of chronic illnesses.

As a result of these changing circumstances, the focus of medical attention is now shifting from the under-nutrition end of the spectrum to over-nutrition in pregnancy, since this too has health consequences for both mother and fetus. Excess fat generates inflammation. During pregnancy, being unhealthily fat (with a BMI over 25) increases the mother's own risk for high blood pressure (pre-eclampsia) and high blood sugar (gestational diabetes). Overweight mothers are also more likely to have 'large for gestational age' babies who are at greater risk of future overweight and future type 2 diabetes in adulthood.[19] Maternal obesity and type 2 diabetes have also been associated with an increased risk for the infant of heart disease.[20] In fact, both extremes of high and low birth weight are associated with dangerous fat around the major organs and an increased risk of future type 2 diabetes and cardiovascular disease.[21]

The mother's diet during pregnancy plays a part in this. If she eats a diet based on getting a fast hit of sugar to generate energy, whether from refined white bread, rice and pasta or from processed foods, her fetus may end up sharing her high blood sugar levels, which increases the child's risk of becoming overweight.

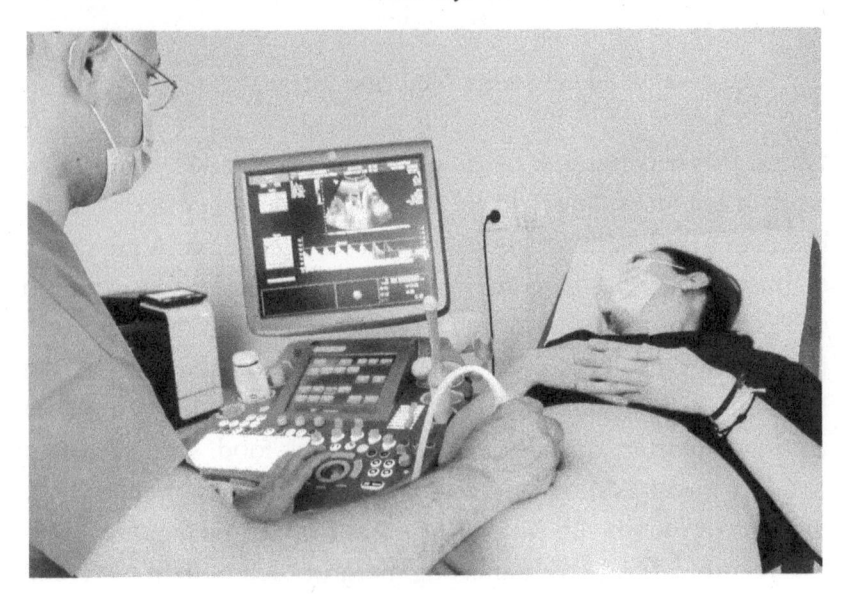

A pregnant woman having an ultrasound scan

(Her infant is 82% more likely to be obese by the age of five to seven than children of women with normal blood sugar levels during the pregnancy).[22] Another, less well researched possibility (so far only demonstrated by research with rats) is that this early exposure to high blood sugar levels programmes the fetus to love sugar and even to be addicted to it, by affecting the reward systems in the brain.[23]

However, the risk of obesity is not just about sugar and white carbs. A 'high fat diet' is often implicated in obesity too. Despite that, an obesogenic diet is not necessarily about eating *more* fat, but about eating too much of the *wrong* fat. One major pathway to obesity is a diet with an unhealthy balance between omega-6 fatty acids and omega-3 fatty acids. This is particularly worrying since the typical Western diet is thought by some to have a ratio of as many as 20:1 in favour of omega-6 foods.[24]

Omega-3 (EPA and DHA-derived) fatty acids are associated with the eating habits of the well-off middle classes, who choose foods like fatty fish (sardines, tuna and especially wild salmon), obscure nuts and seeds, like walnuts and flax seeds, edamame beans and even the bitter-tasting cruciferous vegetables like kale or broccoli disliked by many children and famously rejected by former American president George H. W. Bush. Omega-6 fatty acids, on the other hand, have been cheap and abundant since the late 1950s, when the production of vegetable oils, like sunflower oil, corn or soya oil, took off. This was partly in response to the growing belief at the time that saturated animal fat, such as butter and lard, was a cause of heart disease.[25] Today, omega-6 fatty acids are ubiquitous, found in many processed foods, such as crisps, biscuits, margarine and ready meals, and in fried foods, such as battered fish and chips or chicken. Such foods now make up 50% of the average UK diet, while consumption of fresh foods has declined – less than two portions a day of vegetables and fibre foods is typical.[26] Once seen as a boon, the growth of such industrially produced foods high in omega-6 fatty acids promised a cheap and convenient source of calories so no one would go hungry. But it has turned into a curse, now at the heart of a health crisis, since this unhealthy over-dominance of omega-6 tips the body into an irritable, pro-inflammatory state where it is ready to treat excessive nutrients as if they were pathogens – primed to trigger an inflammatory reaction. This is particularly likely in obese adults whose excess fat itself generates inflammation.

When this unbalanced omega-6 dominant diet prevails in pregnancy, this not only increases the offspring's own risk of obesity, but may have other effects on the fetus. In some recent studies, it has been linked to future behavioural difficulties. One Spanish study examined the blood in the umbilical cords of newborns and found that those who already had a higher omega-6: omega-3 ratio at the very start of life had an increased risk of showing symptoms of ADHD by the time they were seven years old.[27]

However, our obesity crisis doesn't only hark back to a poor diet in pregnancy. Exposure to air pollution during pregnancy also increases a child's chances of growing up obese. In a study of pregnant women in New York City, those who were most exposed to polyaromatic hydrocarbons – created by car emissions and industrial processes – had children with double the risk of obesity aged seven.[28] A similar study in California found that fetal exposure to 'near-roadway' air pollution also resulted in a higher body mass index (BMI) at age ten.[29] However, this growing body of evidence as yet offers no definitive explanation of how and why pollution is associated with obesity.

Stuck with our fat cells

A fetus exposed to its mother's high blood sugar or high levels of omega-6 fats will most likely grow extra fat cells ('adipose tissue') to store the extra energy in the form of fat. Increased fat storage increases its future risk of obesity.[30]

In particular, the period from late pregnancy and into the first year of life, as well as in pre-pubescence around the age of seven,[31] is the prime time for the baby to grow its fat cells (adipocytes) and to lay down fat in preparation for life outside the womb. The number of early fat cells matters as it determines fat mass in adulthood. Kirsty Spalding, a cell biologist working at the Carolinska Institute in Sweden, found that few people first become obese as adults. Although most obese adults have a high number of fat cells, mostly they had been obese as children and had already grown extra fat cells in early life.[32]

A contributory factor may also be a lack of vitamin D in the mother's diet. Vitamin D has a protective effect – it stops pre-fat cells from maturing into fat cells, so helps to keep the number of fat cells down. According to Vaia Chatzi, a professor of preventive medicine, 'Optimal vitamin levels in pregnancy could protect against childhood obesity.'[33]

Once we reach adulthood, the number of our fat cells remains stable; it is only the amount of fat that is stored in them that tends to change. In response to an obesogenic diet, the fat cells we already have may expand to try to store more fat; alternatively, if we eat a more modest and fresh foods diet, our fat cells may shrink because there is less fat to store. But once grown, no diet will get rid of the extra fat cells grown in early life and through childhood.

Even when fat is removed surgically, the body is so efficient at restoring the status quo that it simply grows new fat cells to replace the missing cells, intent on keeping the fat cell number steady.[34]

Stress and fat

A more surprising influence on our potential future weight is our mother's mental well-being during pregnancy. How can a mother's state of mind possibly affect her offspring's weight? For years, psychobiologist Sonja Entringer and her colleagues at the University of California, Irvine, have been exploring this question.

The answer lies in the developmental timetable and in events that take place in the last trimester of pregnancy. In this period, it's normal for levels of the mother's stress hormone cortisol to rise; this is a useful stimulus that enhances fetal brain development and helps its lungs to mature. However, it can have less welcome effects if levels of cortisol are excessively high due to mental and emotional strain, such as suffering a bereavement or traumatic event, or chronic ongoing stress.

While normally there is a protective enzyme in the placenta that can inactivate the mother's cortisol and stop it getting into the fetal bloodstream, very high levels of cortisol can overwhelm this defence and break through. The fetus is then exposed to its mother's high level of cortisol and is likely to be born with a cortisol level that matches its mother's. When this exposure takes place in the last three months of pregnancy, it is associated with a release of blood glucose and in the development of greater numbers of fat cells and increased body fat in the baby's first post-natal six months, increasing the risk of future obesity.[35]

Stressed bacteria

Chronic stress during pregnancy can have other impacts both on the health of the mother and on the future health of her fetus. It can affect the mother's own microbiome – her own unique bacterial ecosystem – which is sensitive to stress. In particular, it can reduce the 'good' bacteria lactobacillus, and can upset the balance and variety of the mother's gut bacteria.

These effects of stress may then affect her baby. The first bacteria to furnish our gut are our mother's – either picked up in the womb (as relatively new evidence suggests) or as we pass through the vagina during the birth process. If her microbiome is not flourishing, our microbiome is likely to be less healthy. This can have a lasting effect as the early months and years of life are critical for establishing a personal microbiome 'signature'.[36] This will be explored further in the next chapter.

You are also what your mother drank, smoked, inhaled or injected . . .

There is also strong evidence that stress drives many unhealthy adult habits and addictions. Often, these habits start as an attempt to manage stress by self-soothing. Whether they are a response to current life stresses, or to the leftover effects of early stress and trauma in childhood, such experiences can both propel people into comfort eating, drug-taking, or seeking other forms of relief or distraction. As Vincent Felitti, professor of preventive medicine, once summed it up: 'Many of our most intractable public health problems are the result of compensatory behaviours such as smoking, overeating, promiscuity, and alcohol and drug use, which provide immediate partial relief from emotional problems caused by traumatic childhood experiences.'[37]

However, when a woman is pregnant this can become an issue for her fetus. The healthy development of the fetus can be damaged very directly when mothers use toxic substances, such as alcohol, nicotine or other drugs. Recent evidence has shown that these substances also affect fathers' sperm, resulting in inflammation that not only lowers fertility but can also pass on damaged DNA to their offspring, increasing the risk of malformations including congenital heart disease.[38] Yet people are so attached to their favourite substances, and they are so much part of our culture, that it has become taboo to challenge their use. In particular, there is considerable resistance to the idea that alcohol is a poison.

'I know, I know . . . I've been cutting down on my drinking. I'm not pregnant yet, Mum. I need to have some fun while I still can.' Last year my daughter's words rang in my ears, and I imagine many people like her feel the same way in a culture where regularly drinking alcohol, smoking, and using recreational drugs is seen as an essential element of creating a playful, non-work mode. Cutting down on consumption is anti-fun; it interferes with the relaxed highs, the pleasurable banter of being part of a group – whether it's a few drinks to unwind with workmates after work, or partying on a weekend with friends. The dilemma is that very early pregnancy matters – but my daughter is also right in thinking that the support she gets from her workmates, and her friends, as well as from her partner, is also a vital part of a successful pregnancy. How then to talk about the needs of a potential fetus without being a puritanical kill-joy? It seems an impossible task.

It's not easy to change our habits. It feels like a cruel deprivation. I have never entirely managed to crack my own sugar addiction, though I can moderate it. Distraction or avoidance can work, but what is most effective is finding alternative sources of pleasurable endorphins, such as physical activity or connecting to other people. Many parents-to-be find the motivation to change their habits once they can picture being with their future baby, start to feel protective of it, and to anticipate that this new relationship will itself be a source of fun and enjoyment.

It is tempting to make light of alcohol use during pregnancy, and to discount those cautious experts who warn that the scientific evidence shows that there is no safe level of alcohol for the fetus. But the issues presented in this chapter show that, across the board, things that we feel our own bodies can cope with are experienced differently by the tiny vulnerable fetus.

The worst-case scenario of excessive alcohol intake is the fetal alcohol syndrome (FAS). This can not only affect the fetus's physical structures as they develop – such as altered facial features with smaller eyes and a thin upper lip – but is also linked to a sensitised stress response and later anxiety as well as a range of learning and behavioural problems. Julia and Simon Brown adopted two such babies without knowing that they had the condition, which is sometimes referred to as the 'invisible disability'. They are now campaigners supporting other people affected by FAS, and have founded the FASD Trust. Knowing what challenges she faced with her children, Julia Brown worries about research that shows that four in ten British women are drinking in pregnancy. As she argues, 'When you're pregnant, every drop you drink, your baby drinks too. When they are born nobody would dream of giving a baby a glass of champagne, yet when you're pregnant and drinking a glass, so is your baby.' In her view, 'There is no safe time to drink.'[39]

Alcohol can indeed have a huge impact on a fetus, especially in the crucial first three months of pregnancy. It's hard to predict the exact degree of individual risk, because many interacting factors are involved: how much alcohol is consumed, how often – and what stage of development the fetus is at. The picture is complex.

Early pregnancy is certainly a particularly vulnerable time. Even when a woman drinks only low to moderate amounts throughout pregnancy, this can produce a negative outcome if it started in

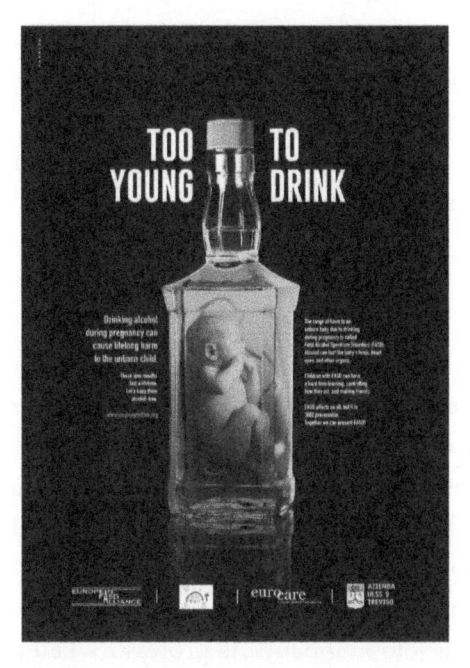

Poster for the 'Too young to drink' international campaign to raise awareness of the dangers of drinking alcohol during pregnancy

early pregnancy, according to research by Californian epidemiologist Gretchen Bandoli. Her work explored the importance of timing, considering if it might be relatively better for the fetus to have little or no exposure to alcohol in early pregnancy even when that is followed by moderate to high alcohol use for the rest of the pregnancy.[40] However, Bandoli's later research stresses that she and her team did not find it was okay to drink alcohol in later pregnancy – she found even low levels of consumption in late gestation were linked to later behavioural difficulties.[41] Vivette Glover, Professor of Perinatal Psychobiology at Imperial College in London, agrees, firmly pointing out that 'the brain develops all through gestation and can be harmed at any time'. There is little doubt that alcohol is one of the leading causes of intellectual disability and has been implicated in children's conduct problems and inattention. This may be due to the impact of alcohol on developing brain structures.

Equally, the common belief that quantity is what matters most and that only large amounts of alcohol are harmful is not supported by the evidence. Professional health leaders who are well acquainted with the research now almost universally recommend no alcohol in pregnancy, to protect the fetus.

Chemical onslaught

Smoking cigarettes is also a well-known major source of ill health. Its effects on a developing fetus can be dire. In the womb, smoking directly exposes the fetus to carbon monoxide. This is a poisonous gas. Once, my boiler flue was blocked up by a builder's rag and the colourless, odourless gas started to build up in my home. It made me feel dizzy, weak and nauseous – not something anyone would wish for their developing baby. As professors Peter Gluckman and Mark Hanson, eminent academics in this field, warned emotively: 'Effectively the fetus of a smoker is chronically carbon monoxide and nicotine poisoned but cannot cry for help.'[42]

In fact, tobacco smoke introduces more than 4,000 chemicals into the baby's circulation. Other poisons include hydrogen cyanide, arsenic and ammonia. Nicotine is also a poison that crosses the placenta and acts as a 'vasoconstrictor', i.e. it reduces blood flow by up to 38%. This deprives the fetus of both oxygen and nutrients. The lack of oxygen has been linked to reduced lung function in infants as well as to lung problems in later adulthood, and sudden infant death. The lack of nutrients can restrict fetal growth and lead to the baby being born small (the more the mother smokes, the smaller the baby) – and raises the chances of pre-term delivery. Smoking, especially in early pregnancy, also increases the risks of heart defects, such as atrial septal defect.

Another way that nicotine affects the fetus is that it, too, raises the mother's own cortisol levels.[43] This may play a part in reducing fetal serotonin, which is linked to later irritability and potential conduct disorders in the offspring, as well as being linked to ADHD. Prenatal nicotine exposure has been strongly associated with future ADHD in many studies, though a recent systematic review disagrees, suggesting that such results may have less to do with maternal smoking and more to do with shared genetics.[44] A couple of intriguing studies have also found an increased risk of ADHD in children whose maternal grandmothers were smoking during their pregnancies with the mothers.[45]

The toxic effects of smoking are very well documented – and this includes second-hand smoking too. Exposure to passive smoking, for example by fathers, may affect babies more even than mothers smoking.[46] One study found a link between fathers who smoke more than twenty cigarettes a day during a pregnancy and their child's risk of asthma.[47] Vaping or nicotine patches are not the solution either, as nicotine itself is toxic to fetal lungs, heart and central nervous system.[48]

Nicotine also activates an inflammatory response.[49] New thinking is exploring the likelihood that smoking in pregnancy has epigenetic effects on the fetus, particularly altering genes involved in inflammation, and that this methylation of DNA increases susceptibility to cigarette smoking-induced diseases[50]

Most people know these facts. There is a hopeful trend towards reduction of smoking in general and in pregnancy in particular. However, as Deborah Arnott, CEO of Action on Smoking and Health (ASH), said in 2018, the 'poorer, more heavily addicted smokers, including those who are pregnant, are not getting the help they need to quit'. When people face a lack of money and resources, and are burdened by stressful responsibilities, living among other smokers, they often become addicted to smoking as a way of coping. If social policies don't find a way to successfully address these everyday realities for many families, the health of many will continue to be damaged.

Individual or social responsibility for the fetus?

Parents and mothers in particular are often given responsibility for the well-being of the next generation, and it is true they do influence the health of the fetus and even its longer-term health outcomes. However, much depends on their own state of health and on factors outside their control. Like the Russian dolls that are nested inside each other, there are many layers of causation, each depending on previous events . . . cells are shaped by their local environment, fetuses are shaped by the placenta and signals from the mother's blood, and new mothers, too, are part of a wider environment – a society that shapes what they can be and do. If they are exposed to pollution, to the stresses of inequality, racism and exclusion, to an unhealthy commercial food environment, there is little they can do single-handedly to protect their fetus.

The fetus shares in the mother's life and her environment, whether she enjoys a tranquil well-nourished existence, or whether her world is violent, unstable or stressed. As a society, we tolerate such radically different starts in life, devolving our own responsibility to ensure the health and well-being of the next generation onto the individual mother, without ensuring that she is supported in this role. Currently, there are no 'rights' to a safe and healthy life for either mother or fetus. Instead, it seems to be easier for the collective to judge the individual woman's mothering behaviours or lack of them.[51]

The extraordinary case of Marshae Jones stirred up these issues in 2018. This twenty-nine-year-old woman was five months' pregnant when she caught sight of the rival for her partner's affections across a car park. She was so enraged with the younger woman that she chased after her, pulling her hair and hitting her. As the younger woman, Ebony Jemison, got into her car, she reached for the gun in her glove compartment and fired it at Marshae. The bullet went into

Marshae's belly. Although Marshae survived, she miscarried her unborn baby.

Jurors in the Deep Southern state of Alabama, USA, took the view that the younger woman acted in self-defence, and exonerated her. Instead, they blamed the baby's death on her mother's decision to start the fight while heavily pregnant, and indicted Marshae for manslaughter. This triggered outrage. In response to such judgements, some women responded angrily that their bodies are their own and that they were being unfairly expected to be 'perfect self-sacrificing mothers'.[52] Ultimately, the Alabama District Attorney decided to drop the charge against Marshae Jones, calling the case 'heart-breaking', taking the view that families on both sides had suffered and nothing would be gained by further legal action. This was an extreme case, which raises many issues about how people understand the relationship between a mother and her fetus. Arguably both women acted recklessly. However, does a mother have a special responsibility to protect her fetus? Can the fetus be seen as separate from the mother? The ethical issues are complex, since mother and fetus are in a relationship like no other. The fetus is part of the woman's body – not yet a separate person, with 'rights', although the US courts are pulling in that direction. Yet as the fetus becomes increasingly viable or capable of a separate existence, it becomes more obvious that it has its own developmental needs that not only the mother but also the people and society around her may help or hinder.

In the US, the response to women abusing drugs or alcohol during pregnancy is often adversarial and punitive rather than supportive. And yet society does have an interest in what happens during pregnancy and in the well-being of both fetus and mother. The way a new body is formed in the womb already sets the course for future health. As we have seen, many basic physiological systems – such as the way we respond to stress, our tendency towards inflammation, the robustness of our internal organs, and our risk of obesity – are being organised in the womb. Yet because the processes are invisible, they are difficult to acknowledge. And because the later adult consequences of events in the womb are so remote, it is easy to fail to see the connection. Events in the womb may not create trouble for the individual until long after babyhood is passed, often only when the ageing body becomes less adaptable and more vulnerable due to the cumulative wear and tear of life's stresses.

Evidence is consolidating that some of the most worrying and prevalent adult health problems of Western society today are directly related to what goes on in pregnancy. The World Health Organization identifies these problems as heart disease, stroke, lung disease, cancer, diabetes and, notably, depression. Despite being one of the foremost health issues of our time and a leading cause of disability, there has been little discussion of how, for some people, depression may have roots in the pre-natal experience of depressed or stressed pregnant mothers, whose high levels of cortisol have been linked with effects on their infant's brain, such as altered wiring of the amygdala, thinning of the pre-frontal cortex, in particular of the anterior cingulate – all areas of the brain involved with emotional regulation, passing on a vulnerability to depression or anxiety in their offspring which may not become apparent until they reach adolescence and beyond.[53]

More shocking still, unhealthy placentas, whether caused by poor maternal nutrition, infection, smoking or high levels of stress and cortisol, are associated with a wide range of negative future health outcomes. As Thornburg and Marshall sum it up, unhealthy placentas are linked to 'reduced coronary arterial dimensions, low arterial elastin, reduced endowment of beta cells in the pancreas, decreased nephrons in the kidney and changes in brain structure and function . . . The sum of these effects leads to increased vulnerability for heart disease, diabetes, stroke and obesity for the remainder of an individual's life'.[54]

These 'non-communicable diseases' or NCDs are increasing at a rapid rate. For example, from 1990 to 2019, the global number of deaths due to cardiovascular diseases increased by 6.5 million people, rising to 18.6 deaths, despite improvements in treatment.[55] Obesity has also soared – currently, approximately 41% of adults and 20% of children and adolescents in the US are obese, while in the UK, most recent figures from the House of Commons suggest 26% of adults and 24% of ten-year-old children are obese.[56] It seems strange that, despite much hand-wringing about the rising obesity epidemic, there is so little public discussion of how early experience may negatively affect many body systems and increase the risk of chronic illnesses, such as cancer and type 2 diabetes (another condition that has also increased at a shocking rate, up by about 60% in the UK over the decade since 2005).[57]

Given these facts, the lack of financial investment in pregnancy care is surprising. Although many policy documents nod to the importance of prenatal care, and there are signs that recognition of its importance is improving, it remains the poor relation in terms of funding. In the UK, spending on maternal care (such as midwives, obstetricians, health visitors and perinatal mental health specialists) has been dropping. It was only a miserable 2.5 % of total NHS spending in England in 2018/19 and has even declined since then to 2.33% in 2019/20.[58]

None of this is an invitation to police women's bodies or to demand that they become 'perfect self-sacrificing mothers'. It is about taking women's health and well-being seriously, acknowledging the crucial role they play in the health of the next generation – while recognising that the wider social conditions in which people live also have a profound influence on the health of the new people coming into existence. These factors will continue to have a bearing on the next influential stage of development, the post-natal years.

Fortunately, there are opportunities to restore and re-set some of the systems that may have not had an ideal start, in the next phase of life – the protective post-natal cocoon.

5.
The post-natal cocoon

'Rock-a-bye baby on the tree top
When the wind blows the cradle will rock;
When the bough breaks the cradle will fall,
And down will come baby, cradle and all.
Oh rock-a-bye, rock-a-bye, mother is near
Then rock-a-bye, rock-a-bye, nothing to fear . . .'

Nineteenth-century lullaby

Many years ago I was working for a dynamic, inspiring man who ran a film company. We were having a drink at the end of the working day when I enquired after his wife and new baby and asked what the baby was like. He bluntly responded that he found babies boring – he would start taking an interest when the child could talk or kick a ball. He was being knowingly provocative, yet in practice his attitude was probably not that different from prevailing views in the wider culture.

Today, the culture has decisively shifted towards a more egalitarian idea of parenting. More mothers of babies are working and more fathers are involved in baby care. This has made early parenthood more visible. Yet despite the increased visibility of babies, babyhood remains a specialist concern, largely for parents and experts, not for society as a whole. There is still some discomfort with making babyhood the subject of public discussion and there is little political engagement with the question of what babies need from adults to flourish. Yet we should be asking these questions, as infancy – like the prenatal period – lays the groundwork for our long-term health.

One reason for this lack of awareness of the role played by very early development may be that babies seem so different from our grown-up selves. At some level, they are a challenge to our view of ourselves. Being in touch with babyhood means being aware of the hugely dependent state in which each one of us begins (and ends) life – not the tough, self-sufficient ideal endorsed by business and politics. In our stressful, adrenaline-driven culture, the dominant focus is on how individuals can get more money and achieve new feats, and how the economy can 'grow'. Ours is a culture that values independence, and which allows little recognition of the vulnerability of our bodies and emotions – or for our protective, animal instincts.

Picture a mother duck, for example, ambling in a relaxed fashion along the riverbank, her ducklings waddling behind her. Suddenly, a large black crow lands in front of them. He hangs around looking menacingly at the ducklings as his potential dinner. He moves towards the mother and her brood. She retreats, moving her ducklings into a defensive, tight-knit circle. The crow continues to move towards them. As he gets closer, the mother duck lunges at the

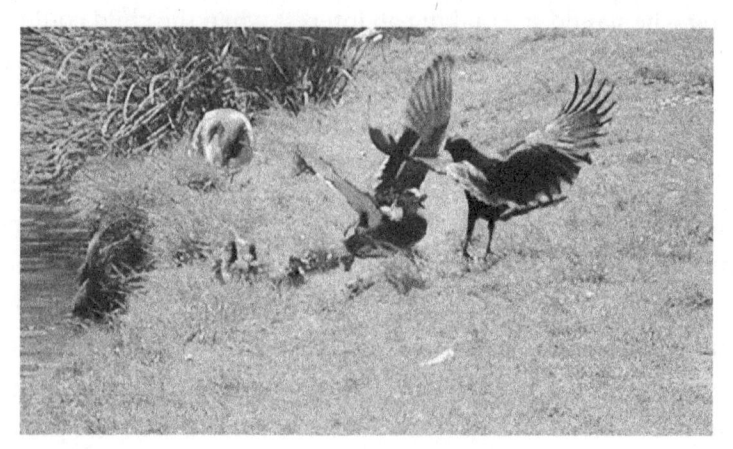

The protective instinct: a mother duck defending her ducklings from a crow

crow, and does everything in her power to protect her babies. This is the basic format for survival: fight or flight, protection of the young. The same behaviour can be seen in other mammals from rats to elephants to gorillas. And humans are no different. We have the same protective urges and desire for our offspring to survive and flourish.

But human infants are more vulnerable than ducklings, who can at least potentially feed themselves and run away from danger. Our babies survive only if an adult takes care of them twenty-four hours a day; no wonder the baby watches closely and tries to keep the attention of the adults who smell familiar, who sound familiar, and who respond to their needs. In the language of attachment research, it is the parents' 'sensitive' and 'responsive' care that protects the baby and supports his or her development. Although providing such attentive care is demanding for the caregiver, it is usually highly rewarding, as, for many parents, this connection with their baby feels intensely absorbing and sensual. The parental urge to touch and look and hold can be compelling.

Yet, until relatively recently, when it has become more common for actresses and influencers, supermodels and singers to post beautiful images of themselves breastfeeding, our popular media rarely celebrated this kind of protective love. Instead, a common tabloid narrative was the desire for mothers to 'get their lives back' after giving birth, and to show their bodies had returned as fast as possible to sexual attractiveness. This often went along with an antagonism to mothers' close physical connection to their babies, especially making others aware of breastfeeding outside the home – not so long ago, the *Express* newspaper crudely described it as 'like urinating' in public.[1] The harsh language suggests a real hostility to the intrusion of caring into the adult world of sex and commerce. However, neither idealisation nor denigration has much to do with the needs of the baby. Whatever narratives about infancy prevail in wider society, babies themselves are focused on survival.

Getting systems up and running

For the human baby, establishing a relationship that provides a protective cocoon is no incidental feature, but a biological necessity. The newborn baby is not yet fully fledged. He or she emerges from the underwater world of the womb onto dry land, not yet a viable individual. The human baby is still dependent on others to nourish him and shelter him from stress, disease and other threats while his or her incomplete physiological (and psychological) systems mature and adapt to his or her social and physical environment. Adult parents provide the supportive context that enables this to happen. The adult, in effect, 'covers' for the immature human, providing many necessary functions until the baby's own systems are fully up and running.

In the womb, basic structures, organs and tissues have grown. But a major task of the months and years following birth is to develop further the regulatory systems that link different parts of the body and

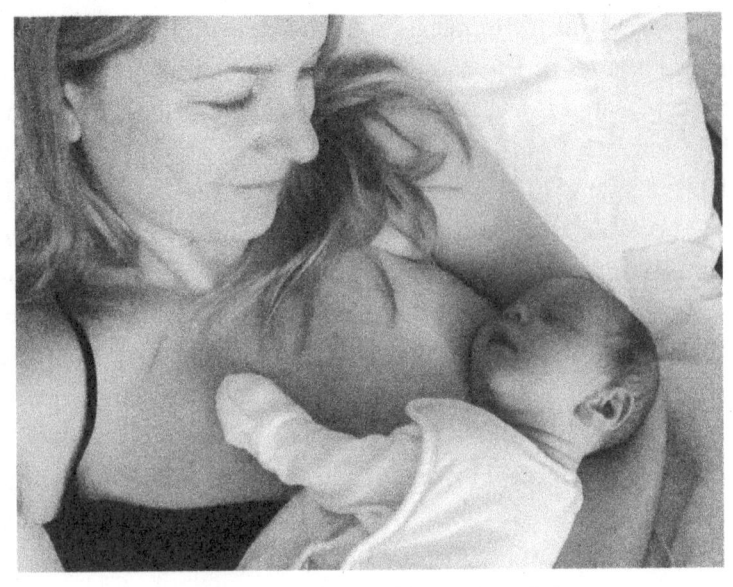

A relaxed mother with her newborn baby

that defend and manage the body as a whole. The aim of these whole-body systems – such as the immune system, vagal system, stress responses, relational systems, with the brain as master regulator – is to enable the individual to meet the physical and social challenges our environment presents, and to sustain health and well-being.

Although they have different functions, these systems often interact and overlap, making it difficult to describe clearly how they work independently. The body is an intricate network of mutual influences, which use common biochemicals to communicate across the body. As Sara Johnson and her paediatric colleagues put it, 'the brain, endocrine and immune systems share a common language of hormones, signalling molecules, receptors and neurotransmitters, which facilitates communication across the network to maintain homeostatic balance'.[2] This chemical language crosses from one system to another, affecting many varied physiological processes. For example, oxytocin plays a role in both blood pressure and cardiovascular health; while serotonin both protects against anxiety and supports brain development.

The first six to twelve months of our lives are particularly important in getting many of these regulatory systems going. But their healthy development is not automatic. Instead, it is shaped by the kinds of experiences we have in these early months – for example, whether we feel safe or unsafe, whether we are breastfed or not, the kinds of bacteria to which we are exposed. In particular, the quality of nutrition and the quality of relationships both have a strong impact on current and future health.

Early nutrition – what's in the milk?

Milk, of course, is our first food, and essential to sustain life – whether we get it from cows or humans. As children's author Maurice Sendak's Mickey joyfully put it: 'I'm in the milk and the milk's in me. God bless milk and God bless me!'[3]

However, there are many differences between human breastmilk and the predominantly cow's milk products known as 'formula' milk. Breastmilk is more than just nutrition. It is a living fluid. Its contents constantly adapt to the needs of the infant, even on a daily basis. For example, if the baby has an infection, the mother's breast milk generates more white blood cells and antibodies to protect her baby.[4] Another extraordinary phenomenon is that breast milk provides a high level of protein in the first couple of months, since that is what the newborn requires, but as that need declines from about two months old, protein levels in the breastmilk also drop. (Formula milk, on the other hand, is inflexible; its high level of protein doesn't change).

Breast milk provides a whole range of invaluable protective substances that support optimal human development and health. Among other things, it supplies the cholesterol and DHA omega-3 fatty acid that are important for brain development. Both are key ingredients in creating firm walls around brain cells, as well as being an important component of the synapses that connect neurons to each other. While omega-3 is now routinely included in formula milk, it is less easy to add cholesterol and other key elements of breastmilk. Most significantly, formula milk cannot pass on the mother's immune antibodies, or her unique bacteria, both of which play a key role in the development of our immune system.

The importance of bacteria

As soon as we are born, we encounter a world swarming with bacteria, viruses and fungi. Within hours they are colonising our body. Before long, there will be as many bacteria as there are cells in our body,[5] mostly found in the intestine and on the skin. At the start, our gut will contain quite a mixed bag of bacteria, including many challenging bacteria.

However, babies who are breastfed receive the bacteria in their mother's milk, which helps to create a more benign 'microbiome' or personal collection of bacteria. Acting as 'pioneer' bacteria – a sort of bacteria starter pack – the mother's bacteria help to establish a microbiome in which potentially good or at least non-harmful bacteria (sometimes known as 'commensals') predominate. This is partly achieved through a substance in her milk known as oligosaccharides – hard-to-digest sugars, which are the optimum food for the protective and beneficial bifidobacteria. While the baby is being exclusively breastfed, these bacteria come to dominate the baby's gut. Bifidobacteria offer protection against pathogens in this early vulnerable period. They may also possibly contribute to managing stress. At least in lab animals, they have been found to reduce anxious or depressed behaviour. There is some evidence for similar beneficial effects in humans, but findings are much more tentative and contradictory. Some small studies have shown that lactobacillus and bifidobacteria can lower the stress hormone cortisol,[6] although a more recent meta-analysis found they only reduced 'subjective stress', but did not have a statistically significant effect on cortisol.[7]

Formula milk and bacteria

Babies fed on formula milk are less well defended against pathogens. Characteristically they have less protective bifidobacteria and a wider range of challenging bacteria at an earlier age – especially more 'bad' bacteria associated with inflammation.[8] Babies fed formula milk tend to have increased baseline levels of pro-inflammatory cytokines. Bottle feeding even one bottle of formula a day in the first week of life is enough 'to alter the infant gut microbiome in favour of pro-inflammatory taxa'.[9]

Unfortunately, giving mostly breastfed babies even small amounts of 'supplementary' formula milk can also prematurely end the dominance of these protective bacteria. It rapidly turns their gut microbiome into one more typical of formula-fed babies. Yet this potential down-side of mixed feeding is not well known and when put forward is increasingly liable to be resisted. For example, this post on Mumsnet:

> My sister was told something similar by her health visitor and was so upset by it. She had struggled and struggled with breastfeeding and was topping up with formula, and the health visitor told her she was negating any of the benefits of breastfeeding by using the formula. I think I would have thrown the HV out of the house if I had been present. Any breast milk is good, and formula is not poison and not going to cancel out the benefits of the breast milk. In my opinion combination feeding can be the best of both worlds.[10]

Certainly, in Britain, exclusive breastfeeding is becoming a minority activity – in 2010, only 17% of mothers were still exclusively breastfeeding their babies at three months old.[11]

Some formula milk manufacturers have tried to tackle the lack of bifidobacteria caused by consumption of their products by enriching them with prebiotics – adding a couple of synthetic oligosaccharides. These formula milks have successfully raised the bottle-fed baby's bifidobacteria closer to the level of a breastfed baby, though this only works if the baby is exclusively bottle fed.[12] However, even this adapted formula milk is still dramatically different from complex, dynamic human breast milk, which offers the baby over one hundred and fifty oligosaccharides.[13]

The heightened immune protection offered by bifidobacteria seems to be most essential in the first few months of life. Once solid food is introduced, greater bacterial diversity starts to be regarded as a good thing and a lack of diversity as unhealthy or 'dysbiotic' – a condition where there are too many 'bad' bacteria and not enough 'good' bacteria, or just not enough varied bacteria.[14] Bacterial diversity naturally increases as the baby becomes more mobile and is exposed to a wider environment, from which he or she can pick up a range of bacteria – from the objects and toys he puts into his mouth, from affectionate visitors who cuddle and kiss him, to the family pets, the carpets and furniture, and from crawling around on mud or grass outside. By the end of the first year or two, the toddler's personal microbiome begins to look more like the more complex and varied adult microbiome, with more than a hundred different species of bacteria (mostly concentrated in the last five feet of the gut, in the colon).[15] Once the microbiome is established (by the age of three), it tends to remain stable, although antibiotic use or major changes in diet, as well as ageing, can affect its composition.

Bacteria and the immune system

One possible explanation for the central importance of bacteria in mammalian health is that the immune system likely co-evolved with the microbes around us. Ted Dinan and John Cryan, leaders in this field for many years, argue: 'Mammals have never existed without microbes . . . The reality is that we have co-evolved, and we are fundamentally dependent upon our colonisers for survival, as of course are they on us'.[16]

One area of mutual benefit is in the digestive process. Bacteria help humans to digest their food by breaking its fibres down so it can move more easily through the intestine and, in return, they receive 'lodging and feeding benefits', as Antonio Damasio put it.[17] A side benefit of this process is that, as the fibre ferments, it generates substances called short-chain fatty acids (SCFAs). One of these, called butyrate, plays a useful role in the immune system – namely, it helps the body to produce immune cells known as regulatory T-cells (Tregs). These T-cells, which live mostly in the colon, are helpful in suppressing inflammatory reactions. They offer some protection against auto-immune diseases such as rheumatoid arthritis, coeliac disease and type 1 diabetes, as well as protecting against food

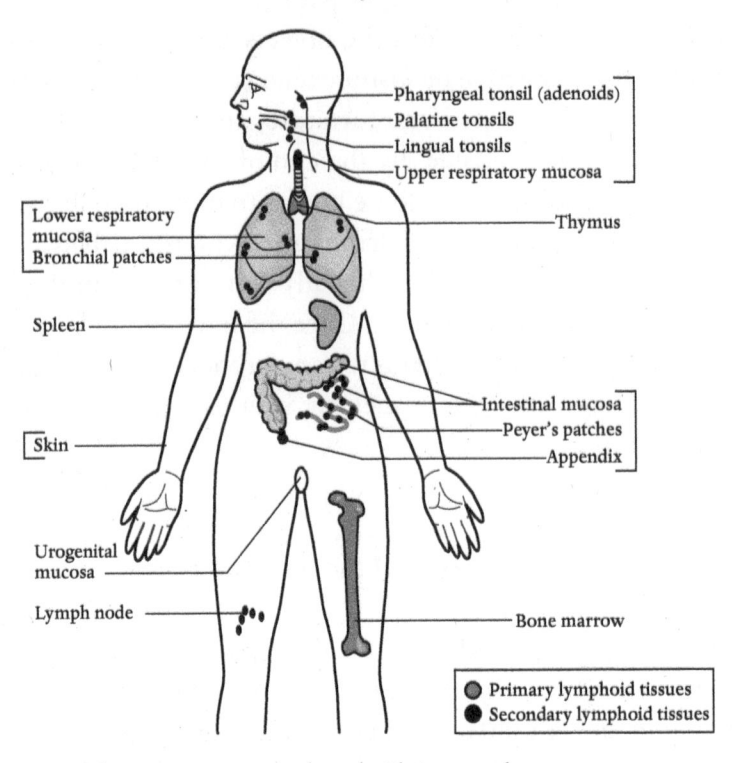

The immune system: lymphoid tissue and organs

allergies and irritable bowel syndrome (IBS).[18] Butyrate also encourages the baby's T-cells to produce the anti-inflammatory cytokine IL-10.

Gut bacteria also help the wider immune system to mature. They support the development of what are known as 'lymphoid structures' (tissue full of white blood cells or lymphocytes), such as the spleen and thymus, as well as the 'Peyer's patches' in the small intestine, which monitor pathogens in the digestive system.

Bacteria also play a role in sustaining a healthy mucus lining to the gut. Although bacteria live around the inner edge of the mucus, consuming the carbohydrates that are present in the mucus – a little like shrimp in a rock-pool on the edge of the sea eating the algae that float there – they also do a useful job of helping to maintain the mucus. As long as they can access plenty of fibre, these well-nourished bacteria will keep producing butyrate, which keeps the mucus nice and thick. The thicker the mucus barrier, the less likely it is that bad bacteria (pathogens) will get through it to trigger inflammation elsewhere in the body.[19] However, when the human 'host' does not eat enough fibre, the bacteria may fill up on the mucus layer for their own nourishment. This can be bad news for the mucus layer: the danger is it degrades and becomes weaker and thinner, which in turn makes it easier for the pathogenic bacteria to get through.

A healthy and diverse gut microbiome underpins the development of many systems.[20] We know this because of studies of what are known as 'germ-free mice', mice deliberately engineered to have no bacteria at all. These experiments have played a significant role in microbiome research, highlighting the role of bacteria by showing what happens without them. There is a range of outcomes, but the complete absence of bacteria particularly affects the mouse's brain biochemistry and neuronal connections, and its capacity to deal with stress. At least in mice without bacteria, the HPA axis stress system becomes unstable and over-reactive, leading to higher levels of stress hormones. As Ted Dinan, professor of psychiatry based at a global microbiome institute, summarised it: 'Resilience to environmental stress seems to be heavily influenced by microbial composition.'[21]

But pathogens are not the only problem for the immune system. Chronically negative and stressful social experiences can also trigger an immune response. Recent research suggests that both emotional trauma and insecure attachments in early life have a physiological impact. The increased stress not only raises levels of baseline cortisol (the stress hormone) but can also raise baseline levels of the immune system's pro-inflammatory cytokines, such as IL-6, TNF and CRP.[22]

One study suggests that very early life is a notably sensitive period for the way that the inflammatory response develops. This intriguing study by Candace Lewis and her colleagues at the Translational Genomics Research Institute in Arizona found that early difficulties in the relationship between a mother and her baby could play out in changes to the baby's immune system. The factors that made a difference were a mother's lack of emotional availability and responsiveness to her baby in the first year of life (but not later, even at age two-and-a-half). This triggered epigenetic processes, silencing genes that regulate inflammation. Their study is particularly significant as it controlled for genetic confounds, using twins to show that the differences in health outcomes in later childhood were 'environmentally driven'.[23]

Such early alterations to the inflammation genes may be long-lasting. One recent study found that the shorter the duration of breastfeeding in infancy, the higher the adult's level of inflammation will be in later life (as shown by the level of 'c-reactive protein' (CRP), a marker for inflammation). This is significant for adult health, as high inflammation levels are associated with a range of illnesses often encountered in later life, including cancer, kidney disease, diabetes, obesity, cognitive decline and depression. In particular, a high level of CRP has been strongly linked to an increased risk of cardiovascular disease, though inflammation is not necessarily its cause – more likely, one of many factors that are involved in the process.[24] In fact, the protective effect of breastfeeding on later CRP levels in young adulthood is 'comparable, or larger' than taking statins, the ubiquitous medications that lower both 'bad' cholesterol and CRP: babies who breastfeed for six to twelve months have around 39% less CRP as adults, while the statin drugs also reduce CRP in adults by a similar amount.[25] How extraordinary then that our media has adopted statins so enthusiastically yet is often so reluctant to speak up for breastfeeding.

At any age, problems arise when the inflammatory process doesn't work effectively and challenges to health are not quickly resolved and healed. When infections become chronic, such as in persistent gum disease or recurring ear infections, or in overweight people

The post-natal cocoon

whose excess fat releases a 'low hum' of inflammatory cytokines, inflammation can turn from a useful and necessary short-term defence against illness to an actual cause of illness and chronic dysregulation.

Clearly, optimum functioning of all these overlapping regulatory systems depends strongly on two things: nutrition that supports a flourishing microbiome, and warm, protective parenting that buffers the child from stress. These two things are, essentially, the foundation of health.

As I research my own condition, Parkinson's disease, I see many of these themes recurring. Scientists exploring its potential causes have recently highlighted the potential impact of early stress, poor early nutrition, poor gut bacteria and chronic inflammation. One route to Parkinson's is thought to be via gut inflammation, which eventually leads to alpha synuclein protein forming clumps in the gut. These clumps then travel up the vagus nerve to the brain where they kill off dopamine neurons.

This fits with the little I know about my own early life. It seems likely that my infant microbiome was unhealthy from the start. I was given a diet of 1950s formula milk, probably made from condensed evaporated milk with added sugar. From toddlerhood, this was followed by the constant presence in my early years of a 'pacifier' in the form of a baby bottle filled with Ribena: the blackcurrant squash again full of inflammatory sugar. I was also frequently separated from my mother very early on (a potent source of stress for an infant).

Each of these factors has been known to reduce levels of soothing bifidobacteria and lactobacillus, and can lead to a weakened mucus layer, an unbalanced gut microbiome and heightened gut inflammation – a state now thought to be a potential cause of the distressed infant crying known as colic, which was indeed a feature of my own infancy.[26] At the time, there was no awareness of this link.

Early immune system

These early months of life are also a vulnerable time for health and survival because many aspects of immune defence are not yet fully functioning. The slippery mucus barrier that stops pathogens getting through the thin wall of cells that line the gut is 'still inadequate',[27] while the inflammatory defence is not yet working at full capacity as it takes much of the first year of life to get up to speed.[28] This leaves the baby relatively undefended from any 'bad' bacteria or viruses that have successfully got past the barriers of skin, stomach acids and mucus to cause infection. In the normal inflammatory process, cytokines orchestrate the concerted action of immune cells such as neutrophils, natural killer (NK) cells, dendritic cells and mast cells, which kill off the pathogenic bacteria. They achieve this by engulfing the bacteria and eating it, followed by repairing the tissue and cleaning up the debris. However, a new baby has relatively few white blood cells of its own, and the NK cells that target viruses also take around three months to reach an adult-like state of function, so, at the start of life, the baby's inflammatory response is underpowered.[29]

Breastfeeding and immune system

However, there is a way to protect the young infant before his own immune system is fully functional. As well as receiving some protection from bifidobacteria, the breast-fed baby gets direct immune support through his mother's milk. One way this happens is through the innate lymphoid cells (ILCs) in the milk, which provide 'frontline immune protection' and help form the baby's mucus layer.[30] Another form of assistance from her breast milk is that the baby also gets to borrow his or her mother's own antibodies for a short time – they provide a sort of 'preliminary immune system'. Through this form of 'passive immunity', the antibodies in his or her mother's breast milk can offer direct protection against some specific diseases the mother's body has already encountered, or against which she has been vaccinated in pregnancy, such as measles, rubella, whooping cough and tetanus.

Each infant's immune system develops differently. For example, as a child, I succumbed to an extraordinarily long list of illnesses: measles, mumps, scarlet fever, German measles, whooping cough, chickenpox and chronic tonsillitis. Although these illnesses were more common in the 1950s before the spread of effective vaccination, my immune system did not seem to be very robust – and possibly the fact that I was not breastfed had something to do with it. 'There's a developmental shape to the immune system that we don't often consider', reflects Dr Dennis Hartigan-O'Connor, a microbiologist at the University of California (Davis) and co-author of an important paper on the different immune systems of breastfed and bottlefed monkeys.[31] 'It's dramatic how that came out in this study. There's a lot of variability in how both people and monkeys handle infections, in their tendency to develop autoimmune disease and in how they respond to vaccines.'

Breastfeeding makes a difference to the baby's own developing immune system, particularly to the 'acquired' immune system, which targets the particular infectious pathogens it encounters over time. Compared to babies fed formula or who are partially breastfed, babies who are exclusively breastfed for at least the first four months have a larger thymus, the gland behind the breastbone that produces immune T-cells. There are a variety of T-cells. Regulatory T-cells guide the immune system to attack only harmful substances and to leave the body's own cells alone. 'Helper T-cells' (Th17) generate antibodies that attach themselves to the invasive virus or bacteria, until other kinds of T-cells – known as Killer T-cells – can reach it and destroy it. Over time, a 'library' of pathogens is created, with data stored for decades by specialist 'memory T-cells', which enable the body to react quickly to the pathogen next time it is encountered.[32] Breastfed babies have both more helper T-cells (Th17) and more robust populations of memory T-cells.[33] Recent research has found that breastfed babies also produce twice as many regulatory T-cells.[34] Perhaps due to this boosted immune system, breastfed babies typically have fewer infections such as gastroenteritis, respiratory illness and ear infections. They are also better protected from nastier, potentially fatal infections, such as neonatal sepsis and the evil-sounding necrotising enterocolitis; they even have a 36% lower risk of sudden infant death syndrome.[35]

As one of the authors of a Lancet study of 2016 said: 'There is a widespread misconception that the benefits of breastfeeding only relate to poor countries. Nothing could be further from the truth.'[36] The Lancet team's analysis concluded that many babies' lives in high income countries, as well as around the world in poorer communities, could be saved if women breastfed for twelve months or more – and in some cases, women's lives too.

Any amount of breastfeeding leads to a greatly reduced risk of the baby going on to develop type 1 diabetes,[37] while breastfeeding plays a part in preventing obesity, which itself is a risk factor for many serious illnesses. Importantly, it can also protect the child from developing childhood leukaemia – with the most protective effect found for those who were breastfed for nine months.[38] Such breastfed babies have a lower risk of developing type 2 diabetes as adults, as well as lower mortality from cardiovascular disease and respiratory disease, according to a recent large-scale Chinese study (drawing on data from the UK Biobank). Xiaoyan Wang and his colleagues suggest these benefits may arise from a better developed immune system, better microbiome and better regulation of inflammation.[39]

As well as protecting the baby, there are also significant health benefits for mothers themselves in embracing breastfeeding. It has a protective effect against future auto-immune diseases. A study of thousands of Chinese women found that breastfeeding dramatically reduced their own later incidence of rheumatoid arthritis (the longer the breastfeeding, the more effect).[40] Other studies suggest that long-term breastfeeding (longer than thirteen months) also significantly reduces women's risk of ovarian cancer[41] and of breast cancer too, as well as diabetes and heart disease.[42]

The obstacles to breastfeeding

Despite rock solid evidence for the health benefits of breastfeeding, there are many obstacles to establishing this tender early bond. As Professor Lesley Page, leader of UK midwives, has argued, when the process of birth itself is no longer seen as a normal bodily and social event, it can become a medical event dominated by professionals whose thinking is focused on risk and pathology. This makes it harder to give due significance to what Page calls 'relationship-based care', and to focus on supporting the often delicate process of establishing an enjoyable relationship between parents and their baby.

Breastfeeding is also not always easy. There may be physical obstacles that get in the way of the ideal. Mastitis – a temporary blocked duct, which stops the milk flowing freely – is painful, and some babies have difficulty latching on to the breast effectively or have conditions, such as upper lip or tongue tie, which need to be fixed first. Some mothers have unusually small, retracted or large nipples, which can make it more difficult. The baby's or mother's illness may get in the way. Sometimes it just doesn't work out. However, the most common reason mothers give for stopping breastfeeding in the first week is the mothers' fear that they had 'insufficient milk'. This is rarely the case (less than 5% of mothers have insufficient milk for medical reasons). However, breastfeeding often needs encouragement to get it established. Support from the people around her and from wider social attitudes – as in the message from the owners of this pavement café in Copenhagen (see picture) – is also essential to enable a mother to take the time to establish the rhythm between

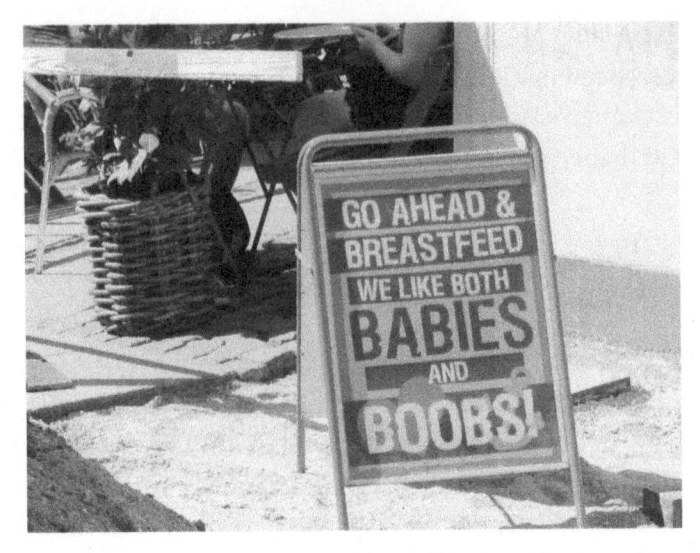

Sign seen on a pavement outside a café in Copenhagen, 2018

her and her baby and to establish a pleasurable breastfeeding relationship.

There are many other factors that can get in the way of the relationship between parent and child – premature birth, disability, an unhappy relationship between the parents or other difficult circumstances. The actor Brooke Shields has written about her experience of having a baby, which was fraught with difficulties – it had been difficult to conceive, the birth was challenging, the baby had a hip problem, and she was also grieving the recent loss of her own father. Yet in many ways the biggest problem was her difficulty in relating to her baby. Her idealised expectations that she would feel an intuitive instant bond with her baby did not materialise. Instead, she says, 'all I felt was distance and dread. Nothing was as I had pictured it'. This made her feel helpless, incompetent and full of self-loathing.

The situation slowly turned around as she learnt to tune in to her baby's communication. As she became more receptive to what her baby was telling her, she began to build a real relationship with her: 'I began to know when she was tired vs when she was hungry or bored . . . I could tell Rowan's mood by the tone or cadence of her cry ... I felt less hopeless.' The baby 'got cuter' as she began to realise Rowan loved being close to her. A turning point was when Rowan refused the bottle of expressed milk offered by Brooke's powerful and dominant mother, but 'quieted down right away' as soon as Brooke took her in her arms. Soon she could not get enough of her.[43] Their unique relationship had taken off.

The politics of breastfeeding

Resistance to breastfeeding used to be mostly a feature of overt male sexism – as expressed by people like the American politician Donald Trump, or by the BBC DJ Alex Dyke, who said on air: 'I blame the earth mothers, you know the ones I mean, the ones with the moustaches, the ones who work in libraries, the ones who wear hessian, the ones they're always on Radio 4 on Women's Hour, they are always pushing the boundaries and making us feel uncomfortable. Breastfeeding is unnatural. It's the kind of thing that should be done in a quiet, private nursery. It was OK in the Stone Age when we knew no better, when people didn't have their own teeth ... but now I just think a public area is not the place for it and fellas don't like it'.[44]

It's easy to dismiss such feelings. However, such cultural hostility is not confined to men. Many women are also uncomfortable with breast-feeding, especially women in economically deprived circumstances. In particular, younger white mothers, and women who smoke, are less likely to breastfeed – 'both a cause and a consequence of deprivation', as Laura Oakley, a British researcher, put it.[45] According to the psychologist Viren Swami and his co-researchers, one reason for this is that economically insecure women face 'greater pressure to treat the breasts as assets that play performative roles, such as in terms of attracting potential partners or to attain material benefits'.[46] Certainly, there is widespread cultural pressure to define breasts in a sexual way, and to live up to idealised images of breasts coming from a consumer society that uses such images to sell a variety of products, including online porn. This affects women of all backgrounds, most of whom are not satisfied with their breasts as they are; however, dissatisfaction is greatest among younger women from disadvantaged backgrounds.[47]

More economically secure and better educated women, on the other hand, who potentially enjoy more sense of agency, are more likely to see their own breasts in active terms. Those who are happy with their breasts and how they look are also more likely to check their breasts for warning signs of cancer and are more likely to want to breastfeed and to maintain exclusive breastfeeding for longer.[48] However, even those who are most likely to breastfeed beyond the early weeks – mainly professional women and black and minority ethnic mothers – do not do so in any great numbers. Only 34% of all mothers are still doing any breastfeeding at six months.[49] Even committed breastfeeders, such as Brooke Shields, can be undermined by a culture that is hostile or indifferent to breastfeeding. When she was struggling, Shields was urged to give up breastfeeding by a powerful trio of her mother, mother-in-law and doctor – they felt she 'needed a break'. However, she instinctively felt that breastfeeding 'was my only real connection to the baby . . . a lifeline', so she carried on.

Most significant of all, the cultural shifts in women's working lives that have taken place in the last few decades have made breastfeeding more difficult. Women from any background may struggle to commit to breastfeeding for practical reasons: most new mothers now face economic pressures to return quickly to work; equally, shared parenting has become an aspiration. These changes raise difficult questions about breastfeeding: how can it fit around work? The recent rise of working from home makes it easier for some mothers to integrate breastfeeding into the working day, but still leaves anxieties about how partners can participate in feeding the baby, especially in sharing the exhausting night feeds.

Britain has become one of the worst countries in the world for breastfeeding. Practically no one is breastfeeding at twelve months (under 1%), unlike New Zealand (44%), Norway (35%), India (92%) – even the USA, with its lack of maternity leave from work, has a better rate of longer-term breastfeeding (35%). Another sign of British governmental indifference to breastfeeding is its abandonment of its annual survey of breastfeeding that had been running for forty years. This matters because breastfeeding for longer than six months is so protective of both the mother's and the baby's future health.

However, the lack of commitment to long-term breastfeeding is good news for the manufacturers of formula milk, whose global sales are heading upwards, and predicted to be a $110 billion dollar industry by 2026.[50] These corporations have successfully changed attitudes with their aggressive and lavish marketing, targeting not only mothers but also health professionals. For example, in 2012, Nestle organised a network of sales people to visit hospitals, doctors, health visitors and community midwives with the aim of developing long-term relationships with them in order to get them 'to support brand endorsement' as well as offering them the opportunity to go on a free three-day trip to Switzerland to hear their corporate messages in full – with a vineyard tour and dinner thrown in.[51] This is presented as a professional collaboration to share scientific information.[52] The food industry's propaganda machine also targets parents, increasingly promoting their milk substitutes through paying influencers on social media, as well as offering apps for chat services and helplines. The messaging can be introduced indirectly. For example, 'Baby Clubs', such as one run by Cow and Gate, which offers parents online advice about bottle-feeding, normalise it as an option: 'There are so many exciting choices in pregnancy. Find out about baby feeding options from C&G baby club, including breastfeeding and bottle-feeding.'

Compared to these well-funded activities, meagre budgets for public health messaging cannot compete. Nor can breast milk be sold to make corporate profit. It is a free, natural, renewable food produced and delivered to the consumer without pollution, unnecessary packaging or waste. Formula milk, in contrast, uses energy in the manufacturing process as well as millions of tons of metal and paper to package (ending up in land-fill), and fuel to distribute; and more than 4,000 litres of water are used to produce just 1kg of formula powder.[53]

Pressure remains to down-play the claims made for exclusive breast-feeding. Perhaps as a result of these pressures, breastfeeding has become a new front in the parenting culture wars. Increasing numbers of feminist journalists and even the National Childbirth Trust (once characterised as archetypal 'earth mothers') have begun to adopt the neutral stance that breast or bottle is simply a woman's choice; they appear to be convinced that differences in health outcomes are relatively 'trivial' or 'negligible', supported by pundits such as the tabloid newspaper columnist Dr Ellie Cannon, who asserts that 'there is an effect, but it's small and I don't believe it poses enough of a risk to be a worry for my patients who do not breastfeed'.[54] Similarly, economist Emily Oster downplays the benefits in her book *Cribsheet*. Although she admits that breast is in fact best 'in terms of infant health', she too questions how substantial these benefits are, given the difficulties that many women experience with breastfeeding. Even Dr Chris van Tulleken, whose work aims to highlight the harms of ultra-processed food, including formula milk, feels that in developed countries it is simply a matter of parental choice: 'If a family decides freely and with the best information to use formula, then it's a good choice in a country like the UK'.[55] What seems to motivate these sorts of argument is less a critique of the scientific findings than a concern that women should not be made to feel guilty if they don't breastfeed.

Of course, inducing guilt is not helpful, and there are many factors that influence parental choices apart from scientific research. Yet perhaps we should question how 'free' such choices are in a highly individualistic consumer culture. Many new mothers find breastfeeding difficult partly because they feel isolated, unsupported and alone with their babies – but they cannot 'choose' to have a supportive community around them if it does not exist. As the Hungarian-Canadian trauma expert Gabor Maté puts it, ours is a culture that has 'lost touch with both the child's developmental needs and what parents require to be able to meet those needs'.[56]

Love, safety and biochemicals

However, breastfeeding is not the only important factor in creating good foundations for health. The quality of the early protective relationships also shapes the important systems that enable us to manage stress throughout life. Parental holding, tenderness and attention all help to create good soothing systems in the baby that will be used throughout life to maintain the body's equilibrium. When the early protective relationships go well, the regulatory systems also flourish.

Whether breast or bottle, the feeding relationship itself, the physical closeness, eye contact and skin contact it brings, has its own health benefits. It reduces stress and anger and generates calming biochemical responses in both parent and baby.[57] It also releases the hormone oxytocin in both baby and parent, which feels good in each.

This hormone, first discovered in 1906, plays a key role in human social behaviour. Oxytocin is involved in social brain networks and supports pro-social emotions, such as maternal care, trust and altruism, while potentially preventing some problems with social behaviour, such as in autism or social anxiety disorder. While the breastfeeding process of the baby sucking and the mother's breast supplying milk is a major trigger for the release of oxytocin, other forms of touch and non-verbal communication – skin to skin contact, affectionate play, stroking, massage and a loving gaze – also release oxytocin. All these forms of physical closeness and emotional engagement generate high levels of oxytocin, and the accompanying relaxed, pleasurable feelings motivate the baby to pay close attention to the vital social cues he needs to read to understand his social world, particularly focusing on looking at and remembering the parents' faces and eyes.[58] Although this continues to some extent into toddlerhood and later childhood, the intensity of communication through touch, facial expression and eye contact declines over time and the level of oxytocin lessens.

Oxytocin itself acts a buffer against stress. Safe in the arms of a protector, feelings of calmness, trust and confidence are generated and fear and anxiety are decreased, enabling 'participation in the world without fear'.[59] One way it reduces anxiety is by reducing activity in the fear-processing amygdala, where there are receptors for oxytocin.[60] It also helps to regulate the stress response by returning the stress hormone cortisol back to its baseline level after a stressful experience.[61] Babies who are regularly hugged and soothed when they need it are more likely to have high levels of oxytocin, while those who are rarely touched or routinely left to cry themselves to sleep may end up with low oxytocin. With less access to oxytocin, they may find it harder to soothe themselves: instead, some learn to deal with stress by switching off and by withdrawing emotionally.[62]

However, this stress-busting aspect of oxytocin only works in the context of a safe, loving connection; children living in neglectful families or who don't feel safe with their parents, don't release oxytocin even when their mothers comfort them.[63] On the other hand, a loving relationship of any kind can trigger oxytocin, as many pet owners can testify.

These early experiences of safety and physical closeness – or lack of it – have lasting effects. They can programme the oxytocin system itself in the first six months of life, leading to permanently high or low levels of oxytocin. Unfairly, there is a risk that those individuals who did not have pleasurable early bonding experiences in their own infancy may then in turn find it more difficult to enjoy their own babies – or, in some cases, even physical closeness in general.[64] Some evidence suggests that this might be the case for adults whose early attachment relationships were of the 'avoidant'

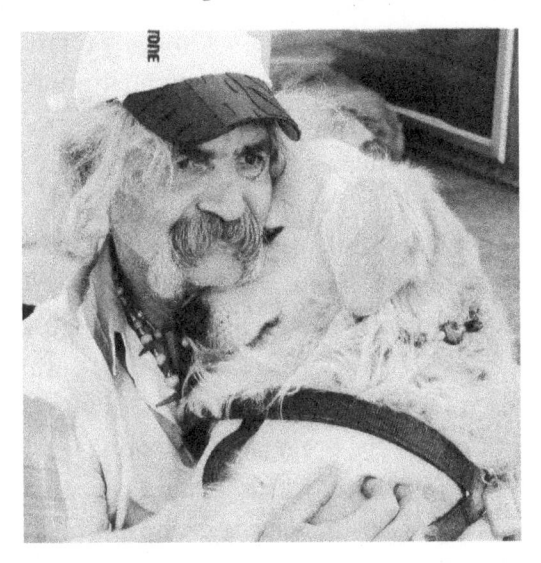

Physically close, trusting relationships, even between humans and animals, can release oxytocin

type, where they had learnt to keep their distance from others at moment of distress; a small study by the Israeli psychologist Tsachi Ein-Dor and his team found such adults' oxytocin genes were silenced.[65]

How the body regulates itself

Although oxytocin plays such a key role in social bonds, it also has effects on bodily functions. Released by the hypothalamus, which is often described as 'the master regulator of the endocrine system', oxytocin also helps to keep many bodily functions stable – from organising sleep patterns to body temperature and blood pressure. It may even have a role in cardiovascular health, since it stimulates the production of nitrous oxide, which expands or dilates blood vessels, lowering blood pressure.

These benefits are mirrored by DHA omega-3 fatty acid, passed to the baby in breast milk (and now routinely added to formula milk, though in much smaller quantities). Omega-3 relaxes the smooth muscle in the walls of the arteries, also potentially improving arterial dilation and reducing blood pressure.[66] A few studies have found a link between lack of omega-3 in early life and high blood pressure in adulthood,[67] but results are inconsistent.

Omega-3 also has the vital function of helping produce biochemicals in the brain, such as serotonin and dopamine, while a lack of omega-3 does the reverse: undermines serotonin synthesis and decreases dopamine release.[68] A lack of omega-3 during early development can even reduce the number of dopamine neurons in the substantia nigra area of the brain[69] – a fascinating fact for people like me with Parkinson's disease, which is characterised by the gradual loss of dopamine neurons in this part of the brain. It might also set up a pro-inflammatory state in the infant brain, which can delay or undermine brain development,[70] though work with baby rats suggests such problems may be preventable as long as the baby's omega-3 is restored during the breast-feeding period.[71] The good news is that, even in later life, omega-3 fatty acids can still help to calm neuro-inflammation, by generating 'resolvins' that decrease inflammation.[72]

Overall, both oxytocin and omega-3 are crucial elements of the protective cocoon in early life – and their effects are overlapping. Both lower blood pressure, reduce inflammation, act as a buffer against stress, lower heart rate and protect the cardiovascular system, as well as potentially reducing anxiety. These benefits are linked to breastfeeding, but can act independently of breastfeeding. So for fathers, trans mothers or adoptive mothers, who want to share the pleasures of feeding, or for those mothers who struggle with breastfeeding for whatever reason, some of the same benefits can be achieved by consciously adopting naked skin-to-skin contact as well as other forms of touch, holding, rocking and mutual eye gazing as part of bottle feeding or just enjoying being with the baby.

The post-natal cocoon

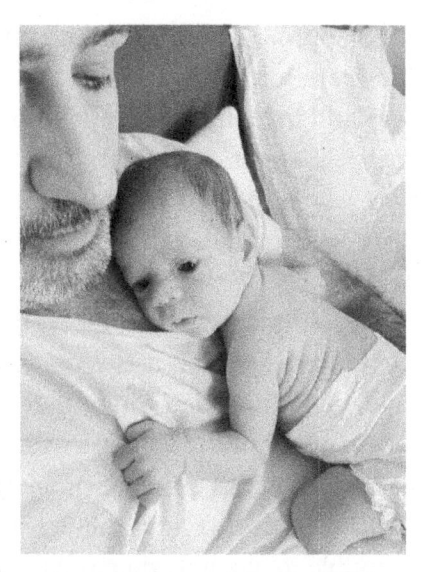

Fathers can also be part of the protective cocoon

Serotonin as emotional regulator

Another key biochemical in the early protective cocoon phase of life is serotonin, a substance that is mostly produced in the gut and which affects many cells in the body. Popularly known as a 'feel good' biochemical, it has some similar functions to oxytocin and is similarly boosted by close, loving physical contact in the early infant period. Levels of serotonin build up most intensely over the first two years of life, and then more slowly until the age of five.

Serotonin doesn't generate the strong positively rewarding feelings that dopamine can produce. However, it helps many systems that are crucial for well-being – such as digestion and the stress response – to function well, and alleviates stress and anxiety by reducing amygdala activity. New thinking suggests that different serotonin receptors have slightly different functions: the receptor known as 1A supports the capacity for tolerance and passive coping with adversity, while serotonin receptor 2A promotes a more active and solution-focused approach to coping with difficulty.[73] Clearly, when serotonin levels are low, both patience and adaptability may be harder to achieve and inattentiveness and impulsive aggression become more likely.[74] A stressful infancy can upset the balance between these two key serotonin receptors and tip behaviour towards the impulsive and inattentive side of the scales.[75]

One highly stressful experience when we are in infancy is the absence of a mother. Experiments with monkeys first suggested that there may be something special about close physical contact with the mother's body in generating serotonin. Baby rhesus monkeys who are denied that close contact, who are kept apart from their mothers and instead reared with a group of monkeys their own age, have lower serotonin than normal and they grow up to be more impulsive and susceptible to alcohol when offered it by researchers as adolescents or young adults during a daily 'happy hour'.[76] Being separated from playmates, on the other hand, has no effect on serotonin levels.[77] The effect of separation seems to be specific to the loss of mother: even when the baby monkey is warmly cuddled by other unrelated adults, his or her level of serotonin stays low, and this tends to persist into adulthood.[78] These sorts of findings about the lasting effect of early maternal absence on the serotonin system have been repeatedly shown in many lab experiments, according to monkey expert Stephen Suomi.[79]

They are also echoed by research with humans, which has showed that children separated in early life from their main caregiver, or who are on the receiving end of aggressive or rejecting parenting, also tend to have reduced serotonin levels.[80] Other small-scale studies have also found a transient depletion of serotonin in new mothers who are depressed, a sadly common experience shared by up to 20% of new mothers.[81]

However, despite wide acceptance of 'the serotonin theory of depression', a recent major review found no consistent evidence that depression is caused by lower levels of serotonin.[82] Many other factors may play a part. Genetic predisposition may be relevant. Lower serotonin levels may be linked to high levels of the stress hormone cortisol, or to long-term antidepressant use. Omega-3 short chain fatty acids (SCFAs) and vitamin D are also necessary for a healthy serotonin system,[83] as are particular gut bacteria such as the clostridiales and staphylococcus.[84]

Vagal nerve and the cocoon

Another system that matures in early life is the vagal system. The vagal nerve is a very long nerve that runs all the way down the body from the brainstem to the gut. It sends its wispy nerve fibres, like etiolated fingers, into many key areas of the body – from the ears, mouth and vocal chords to the heart, lungs, liver, stomach and gut. It is a roving reporter, gathering intelligence about the state of the whole body and transmitting this information back to headquarters in the brain, so that bodily functions can be co-ordinated. At the same time, it acts as a calming diplomatic service, providing strong anti-stress and anti-inflammation properties. It can play a key regulatory role in many bodily functions, from heart rate to the digestive system, and can also help to dampen stress and inflammation.

According to American psychologist Steven Porges, there are two parts of the vagal nerve system, upper and lower. The upper part is involved in social and emotional communication. Its nerve fibres are linked to nerves in the face and larynx, and are activated in behaviours such as listening, vocalising and swallowing; they also reach into the heart, influencing resting heart rate. The lower part of the vagal nerve, on the other hand, reaches down into the digestive system, supporting digestion and food absorption, as well as suppressing unhelpful inflammatory reactions.

In the 1990s, Porges highlighted the interactive nature of the vagal system, describing how the upper part of the vagal system is influenced by early non-verbal interactions between parent and baby, particularly in the first nine months after birth. This is a period during which the upper part of the vagus is rapidly myelinating (improving the speed of its communications). Interestingly, the vagus myelinates on much the same timetable as when brain neurons are myelinating, particularly the neurons in the prefrontal, 'social' brain, with which the vagal nerve connects.[85] While there is some dispute about whether the vagal nerve is involved in eye contact and facial expression,[86] Porges found that this myelination process flourishes best when there is a strong emotional connection between parent and baby, particularly demonstrated through responsive face-to-face contact and soothing touch.

As mothers and babies tune in to each other emotionally, their bodies synchronise: 'both mothers and infants reciprocally adapt their heart rhythms, ultimately forming biological synchrony in the acceleration and deceleration of heart rates'.[87] The baby shows his enjoyment of this mutual attunement by cooing and babbling.

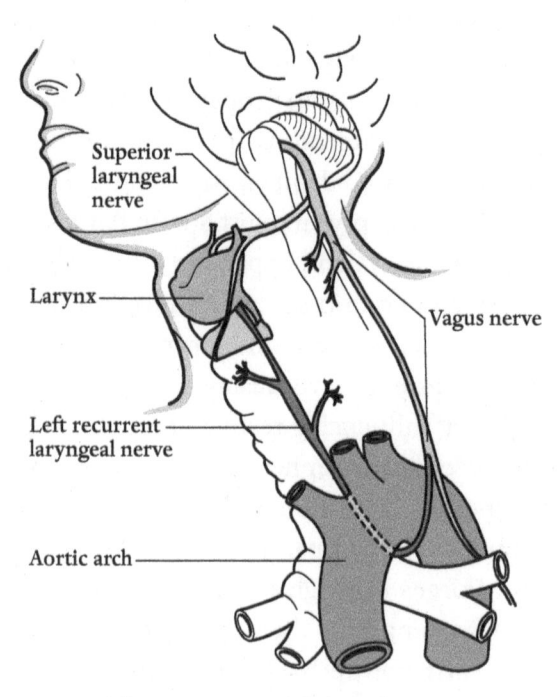

The upper part of the vagal nerve

Even as early as at three months, the more harmonious and well co-ordinated they are, the better the ventral vagal nerve matures and myelinates and sets up a healthy vagal 'tone',[88] which means the baby's vagal system is able to adapt to circumstances by increasing or decreasing heart rate as needed. When the baby does something active, such as sucking or eating, the vagal brake is released, allowing heart rate to increase. But when the baby's body is focused on more passive activities, such as digestion, or recovery from stress, the vagal 'braking system' comes back on, lowering heart rate. Similarly in social situations, the vagal brake can disengage to allow active interaction or can engage to support more calm, reflective behaviour.

One illustration of this is called the Still Face test. In this experiment, the mother is asked to deliberately ignore her baby – the opposite of mutual co-ordinating and synchronising. This is unpleasant to watch, as babies inevitably become distressed. However, those who are used to responsive, well-attuned relationships are better able to deal with it (using their well-myelinated vagal nerve). Their heart rate increases to deal with the challenge of mother's surprising stony expressionless face, then slows down again when the mother restores her attention after two or three minutes, returning the baby quickly to a state of equilibrium. Babies in poorly attuned relationships are less able to manage their distress and recover quickly.[89]

Good vagal regulation as early as two or three months old is associated with social competence in later childhood.[90] It can predict our capacity for emotional self-regulation at the age of two, and even our likely capacity for empathy as an adolescent.[91] One study of teenagers found that those who were securely attached and most empathic were also those with the highest vagal tone.[92] Good vagal tone in adulthood continues to be linked to positive emotions and has a protective effect against inflammation and cardiac risks.[93]

Below the diaphragm, the lower part of the vagal nerve works at a slower speed than the upper vagal nerve, as it is not myelinated. Its branches travel down into the abdomen, via many

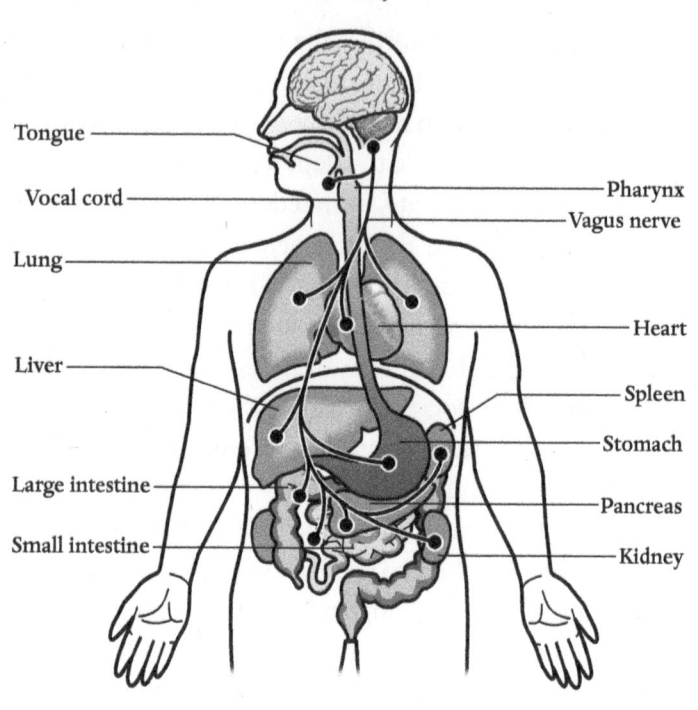

The vagal nerve pathway through the body in relation to the internal organs

significant organs. It reaches into the digestive system in the lower part of the body, where it supports digestion and food absorption, as well as having the capacity to suppress inflammation in the gut by releasing the neurotransmitter acetylcholine.[94]

The lower vagal nerve also responds to the biochemical messages made by gut bacteria, such as GABA, dopamine and serotonin (50% of dopamine and at least 90% of serotonin is made in the gut). Vagal nerve fibres have receptors for serotonin and dopamine and take their messages up to the brain, where they can affect mental states. This is a relatively new way of understanding the links between body and brain. As Philip Strandwitz, a post-doc in Boston, put it: 'We're learning so much about ourselves and the brain is no longer this magical organ in isolation. Instead, it's obviously connected to all facets of our being, and it turns out microbes are part of that.'[95]

The post-natal cocoon

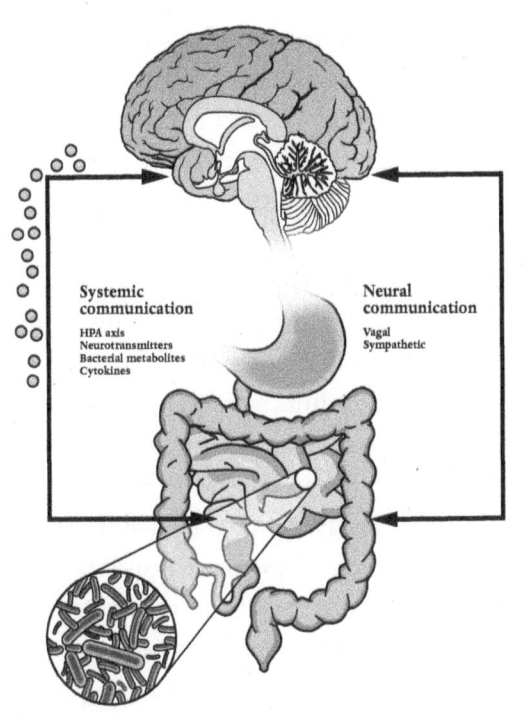

Two-way communication between gut and brain via neural pathways or neurotransmitters

Social self as a regulatory system

Although most of the regulatory systems mentioned so far keep the body functioning in response to basic inputs from the surrounding world, such as food, air quality, or germs, many are strongly shaped by their social context too. Optimum health is derived from the quality of human relationships, particularly in the early protective relationships of infancy, when systems are being set up. However, we also need a dedicated system to regulate our physiological emotional reactions as we participate in the social world and manage the threats and challenges and stresses it throws up.

One way we manage the social world is by developing a stable idea of our 'self' in a world of 'selves'. I believe this baseline sense of 'who we are' is itself another regulatory system first established in early life in response to our experiences. It is partly constructed through our sensory experiences and from the feedback our bodies provide, but it is also constructed from the interactions we have with other people, and the feedback they give us. Other people within our social environment can evoke some potential qualities within our DNA, while other potentials may not emerge.

The way we are 'seen' by others affects our sense of who we are. In infancy, we cannot decide for ourselves that we are lovable, amusing and clever if the adults around us constantly convey their dislike, their contempt for our stupidity and rejection of our humour. If the adults around us are themselves stressed and aggressive, they may encourage us to be 'a fighter' or alternatively might deride us as a 'wuss'. These basic building blocks of the self are established non-verbally from the moment of birth. In fact, parental attitudes that pre-exist our birth can shape our personality. Even if we have the genetic material that might lead to a good-natured temperament or a talent for music, we cannot enjoy or fully develop those potentials in a home that fails to recognise or support them.

This can have a deep impact on our sense of self and sense of autonomy. As the psychotherapist Jean Knox has pointed out, we need to feel we 'have an effect on and produce a response from those around us'.[96] Without a responsive partner, there may be a feeling like a black hole where self should exist. Equally, hostile or dominating caregivers can destroy any feeling of autonomy. There is evidence that over-controlling, intrusive parenting of toddlers – where the adult dictates what the child should feel or do instead of paying sensitive attention to what the child does feel – hampers the child's own ability to learn self-control by the age of five.[97]

Humans are not born independent, nor fully capable of managing their emotional responses. We mature by forming 'regulatory dyads' with our caregiver(s). In a healthy early relationship, the adults do most of the regulatory heavy lifting (as well as literally carrying us) – they regulate and protect us while we learn how to manage our body and behaviour.

Through active parental management, our body learns how to manage stress, challenges, and changing feelings. Vagal tone is established, oxytocin and HPA stress response baselines are set, and the prefrontal cortex develops its ability to put brakes on the emotions generated by the amygdala.[98] With the adults round us, we learn to recognise and name our emotional states, which will help us to anticipate and manage our own reactions and, in time, to predict how other people will react to us.

Self-regulation is something that emerges from months if not years of close relationship. As Steven Porges said, 'as mammals, we evolved to take care of each other'.[99] When this goes well, we gradually develop the 'ability to function independent of other people for short periods', and as we mature, we are able to sustain self-regulation for longer periods. With adult guidance and encouragement, we gradually learn to manage threatening or emotionally arousing situations in constructive ways: we build both the socioemotional skills and the balanced biological systems that can deal with stress. However, although this learning becomes deeply internalised in the way we behave and in how our bodies react to stress, we still need other people's help with regulation. Even in adulthood, we continue to depend on at least a few other people for ongoing support when it is needed, and in old age, those dependency needs increase once again, coming full circle.

So what happens to these overlapping, complex body systems when those early regulatory partners are unavailable or abusive? Or when a child's early life adult partners in regulation are consistently unsupportive or stressed?

PART THREE
When Things Go Wrong

6.

Unprotected: stressful relationships and how they affect health

*'An only life can take so long to climb
Clear of its wrong beginnings, and may never'*

Philip Larkin, 'Aubade'

*'We played dolls in that house where Father staggered with the
Thanksgiving knife, where Mother wept at noon into her one ounce of
cottage cheese, praying for the strength not to
kill herself. We kneeled over the
rubber bodies, gave them baths
carefully, scrubbed their little
orange hands, wrapped them up tight,
said goodnight, never spoke of the
woman like a gaping wound
weeping on the stairs, the man like a stuck
buffalo, baffled, stunned, dragging
arrows in his hide.'*

Sharon Olds, 'The Pact'

More people than we like to acknowledge simply don't grow up experiencing the kinds of relationships that deliver consistent safety, good physical nourishment, attention to how they feel and commitment to their welfare that is love in action. That might seem to be a demanding list of qualities, but each is vital in its own way in producing an emotionally and physically resilient human.

Worse news is that many children suffer from more active forms of harm or from a lack of parenting, yet most societies struggle to acknowledge these realities. It was not until the 1970s and 1980s that the social and cultural taboos that had prevented us from recognising the ubiquity of domestic violence and the existence of widespread childhood sexual abuse began to be broken. Even now, many decades later, such abuse is still being dragged into the light: in the UK, a prolonged government-appointed Independent Inquiry into Child Sexual Abuse finally reported in 2022, acknowledging the extensive abuse of children 'in care' in publicly funded children's homes.[1]

The remarkable American poet Sharon Olds is herself a survivor of sexual and physical abuse at the hands of both her parents. As her poem 'The Pact' (featured at the start of this chapter) vividly suggests, abusive adults who hurt children are often themselves wounded, vulnerable people. In such 'risky' families, a key factor is often that the parents have not learnt to manage their own emotions. As a result, they tend to react without recognising the impact of their behaviour on their children's emotions and sense of self. Their own lack of self-regulation may erupt in the form of anger, contempt and physical or sexual assault, or it can take a more avoidant form, where the child's needs and feelings are ignored and minimised, or where care is disrupted by casual changes in caregivers or by prolonged separations.

Dealing with these issues is my daily bread. They are the familiar but always unique experiences that many clients bring to psychotherapy. Thankfully, therapeutic treatments have become mainstream, and are often effective in mitigating some of the damage. In my own work, this is achieved partly by consciously exploring and witnessing the past with sensitive understanding, but also by cultivating awareness of and support for the client's ongoing development and value as a person. However, undoing the painful devaluations of an abusive childhood is rarely quick or easy. As Sharon Olds once put it in an interview with Kate Kellaway, 'It is a lifelong labour trying to turn away from lies such as that one is worthless.'[2]

What is less recognised is the effect such experiences, particularly in the key formative early months and years, can also have on our body and long-term health prospects. Where a protective parent soothes stress away and guides us in developing constructive coping strategies to manage it, the body's defensive systems, such as immune and stress systems, are also likely to flourish. However, failures of parenting can undermine these defensive systems, leaving our health exposed. Just as with the psychological damage to the sense of self faced in therapy, these early physiological effects are invisible – and may only reap their harvest decades later in adulthood, when health problems start to emerge.

ACES high?

This was first strikingly demonstrated by 'probably the most important public health study you never heard of', as the journalist Jane Ellen Stevens described it – the ground-breaking research of Vincent Felitti and Robert Anda. In her highly readable account, Stevens describes how Dr Felitti came to establish the concept of 'adverse childhood experiences', known as ACEs.[3] In the 1980s, Felitti was working at the Kaiser Permanente Department of Preventive Medicine in California, running clinics to reduce smoking, obesity and stress. After a while, he became puzzled by the fact that just when obese patients were succeeding in losing weight, they would drop out of the programme. He wanted to find out why, so he approached over 200 patients, asking them to help by answering a questionnaire. The task was routine and the questions repetitive; eventually Felitti lost concentration and muddled up two questions together, accidentally asking one woman 'how much did you weigh when you became sexually active?' His patient startled him by answering his botched question with: 'forty pounds'. He was even more shocked when she explained tearfully that she was only four years old at the time and the sexual activity was with her father. As Felitti started to get his head around this, navigating through tricky waters to find a way to ask other patients the right questions, what emerged was a startling revelation that over half of his obese patients had suffered sexual abuse.

However, when he presented his findings to his colleagues at a conference, he encountered general disbelief and rejection, and scorn at his naïveté in believing his patients – not that different from the reaction Sigmund Freud got over 120 years ago, in the 1890s, when he too tried to highlight the prevalence of sexual abuse of children. Unlike Freud, however, Felitti did not turn away from his patients' stories. Instead, he decided to test the evidence. He approached over 26,000 patients from Kaiser Permanente's enormous patient database to participate in a study. Over 17,000 agreed to be recruited.

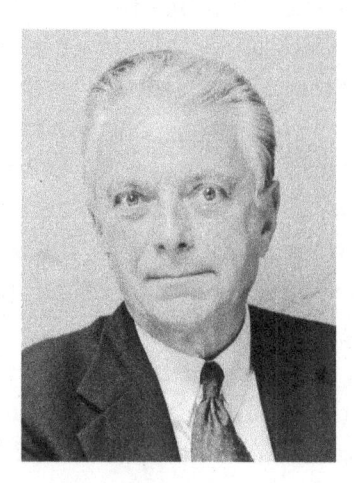

Dr Vincent Felitti, originator of the ACE study, which identified the links between adverse childhood experiences and later health outcomes

He worked with his physician and epidemiologist colleague Dr Robert Anda to develop a new questionnaire about childhood experiences of various kinds, including neglect, which were added to the patients' routine medical questionnaires. The new questionnaire was a radical departure for the medical profession at the time. The underlying question it posed was *'What happened to you?'*

When Felitti and Anda analysed their results, in the mid-1990s, they were stunned to discover how widespread such experiences were: a majority of people in their relatively middle class, and largely white patient cohort had experienced some sort of childhood 'adversity'. At the time, these were defined as experiences of being beaten, humiliated, threatened, sexually abused, physically neglected, emotionally neglected, not being raised by both parents, living with a depressed, addicted or mentally ill parent, witnessing domestic violence or having a parent who had been to prison. No single ACE trumps the others, although Felitti is quoted as saying that chronically being put down or humiliated has a marginally greater impact than the rest.[4]

More ACEs, worse health

Analysing their data further, they made some important discoveries. The more categories of adverse childhood experiences (ACEs) a person had experienced, the more likely they were to suffer serious health problems in adulthood. There was a 'dose-response' effect: the more adversities, the more health problems. More recent work done in the UK has found that as little as one ACE can affect how long you live, while even two ACEs raises the risk for cardiovascular disease, stroke and respiratory disease,[5] as well as for cancer.[6] However, since the start of their work, it has been clear that individuals with a high ACE score of four or more are the most vulnerable to later ill health, with much higher rates of non-communicable diseases (NCDs), such as chronic obstructive pulmonary disease, cardiovascular disease, lung cancer, liver disease and depression.[7]

Such clear links between adverse early experiences and unhealthy ageing were a revelation. Previously, the conventional understanding was that these kinds of health outcomes were due to poor adult lifestyle choices, such as smoking, excessive drinking or drug-taking, and poor diet. In Scotland, for example, a large percentage of the population has a poor diet, and there are high levels of smoking and alcohol abuse; around two-thirds of the population are either overweight or obese. Scotland also has higher death rates from cancer, heart disease and stroke than anywhere else in the UK. But are pies and chips the cause?

Felitti and Anda argued that this was an incomplete picture. Although lifestyle choices (such as diet and smoking) obviously do matter, they are not the whole story. Felitti and Anda were ahead of the curve in grasping that underlying psychological drives also play an important part in drawing people towards addictive eating, smoking or drug-taking. They recognised that, for some, such addictions could be driven by an attempt to self-medicate, to relieve the pain of early mistreatment – or could even be driven by an altered neurobiology set in motion by such negative early experiences.[8]

Today there are numerous personal accounts confirming their thesis, describing these experiences from the inside: books such as Roxane Gay's *Hunger*, which describes how, after being gang-raped by a group of boys when she was twelve, she found herself eating to create 'a protective shield of flesh' and, at the same time, using food to soothe her unbearable emotions.[9] A few academic studies – such as one cross-sectional study observing men and women in prison – have also found that over-eating may indeed be particularly linked to childhood *sexual* abuse, though not to physical abuse.[10]

The ACE model has been influential and maps out the territory in a useful way. It has played a key role in establishing the links between early experiences and later health outcomes, which subsequent research has corroborated. For example, Cristina Barboza Solis and her French colleagues analysed data from a large cohort of British children who had been followed since 1958 well into middle age. This long-term study confirmed that adverse childhood experiences did indeed have health consequences, increasing physiological 'wear and tear' and creating negative impacts on nervous, endocrine (hormone) and immune systems.[11]

With that said, the ACE model is a fairly blunt instrument and has been criticised for being so. It relies on retrospective recall of childhood experiences, which lacks the stringency of prospective studies that monitor the process of change, as it happens, over a period of time. The model also lacks specificity about the age that adverse experiences occur. This is problematic, since timing is important and can shape outcomes, most strongly affecting systems when they are in development.

Most research has focused on early childhood as a category defined only as 'under five'. With this wide focus, it has established strong links between maltreatment under five and later aggressive and depressive tendencies in children. For example, an early prospective study that followed pre-school children through to the age of fourteen found that harsh physical treatment in earlier life led to consistently higher levels of aggressive behaviour, and of depression, than later maltreatment did.[12] More recently, Erin Dunn's retrospective study of 2,892 African-American adults confirmed that being exposed to maltreatment or interpersonal violence, specifically under the age of five, doubles the likelihood of having later depression or PTSD symptoms – compared to children who are exposed to trauma at a later stage in their development.[13] Such early exposures – particularly to violent behaviour or harsh parenting – can have long-term effects, leading to an increased likelihood of suffering from anxiety and depression even in adulthood.[14]

Since then, a unique study by the psychologist Erin Hambrick has begun to drill down even further into the 'under five' category to explore the consequences of stress at different stages of development. Hambrick and her team, under the auspices of the Child Trauma Academy in Texas, found evidence that the perinatal period – defined as the first two months of life, in her study – had the strongest impact on later health outcomes, particularly through their effect on basic systems involved in physiological regulation, such as the stress response, and the ability to manage emotional arousal and appetite. Poor early relationships in these first months, which she called 'relational poverty', were the strongest predictor of negative outcomes for children.[15] Unfortunately, for many parents this period of adjustment to parenting is also a time of increased marital dissatisfaction and conflict, which can affect their babies' stress processing systems.[16]

Relational poverty in the form of physical abuse or severe family stress in early life has also been linked to an increased risk of type 1 diabetes in childhood.[17] Two interesting studies found this to be the case particularly when the stressors occur in the first two years of life.[18] However, not all studies reach the same conclusion: epidemiologist Jessica Bengtsson's study of 2 million Danish children found those who experienced adversities had a 'negligible' increased risk for type 1 diabetes. Nevertheless, she points out that her study did not take account of the age of the child when adversities were experienced; she acknowledges that such experiences during a sensitive developmental period may indeed affect the risk of type 1 diabetes.[19]

ACEs are all about the cumulative harm caused by repeated negative and stressful experiences of often overlapping and different kinds. A different approach is to investigate whether there are links between specific types of maltreatment and particular health outcomes. Several studies have found that harsh parenting – defined as coercive, emotionally invalidating, hostile, humiliating, bullying or physically abusive behaviour – is correlated with a variety of adult ill-health conditions, such as fibromyalgia, chronic fatigue, depression, anxiety, high blood pressure and cardiovascular disease risk.[20]

The mechanism for these links between early adversity and later ill health is usually attributed to the increase in stress hormones and increased inflammation caused by stress.[21] Certainly, abuse in childhood is associated with higher levels of inflammation in adulthood. For example, one prospective study of children under eleven who were followed over thirty years confirmed that physically abused children had an increased risk for raised levels of inflammation lasting into adulthood.[22]

Stress affects the immune system

Felitti was an important pioneer. Yet he was not the only researcher turning his attention to the long-term health impact of childhood stress and trauma in the 1990s. The psychologist Gregory Miller has also been a prolific contributor to psychoneuroimmunology (how the mind affects the immune system) since the late 1990s and is a leading researcher in this field. He is particularly interested in understanding why people respond differently to stress and infection and how psychological stress gets 'embedded' in the body's systems. Its impact on the HPA axis stress response is well established, but Miller's work suggests that the white blood cell macrophages of the immune system can also be 'programmed' or altered by stress.

Crucially, Miller emphasises that it is *early* stress that programmes both the developing HPA axis stress response, and the inflammation-generating macrophages of the immune system.

Both the HPA axis stress response and the immune system are highly 'plastic' in early life; they are programmed or shaped by the circumstances they are exposed to. The two systems – stress and immunity – also affect each other. Described by Californian psychologist Rena Repetti and her colleagues as 'meshed gears', the HPA axis and immune system can both become hyperactive in response

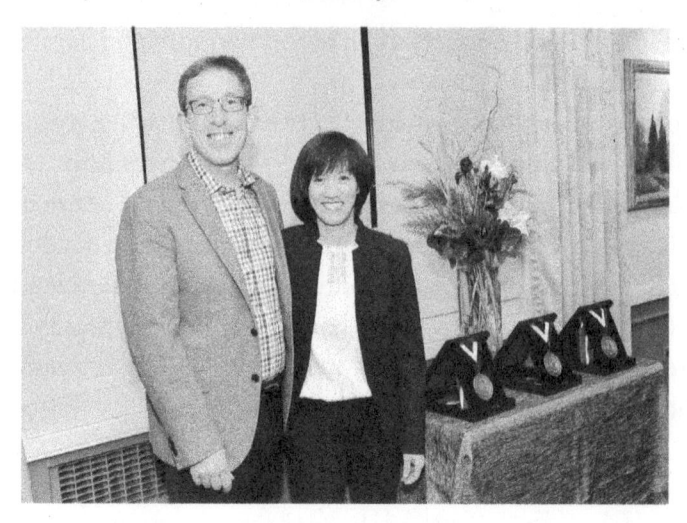

Professors Greg Miller and Edith Chen, life partners and colleagues, whose 'biological embedding' hypothesis explored the links between early stress and later inflammatory disease

to early 'harsh rearing' conditions, offering some immediate protection but long-term health disadvantage.[23]

Under conditions of chronic stress, the immune cells that are constantly exposed to cortisol released by the stress system can end up 'insensitive' to cortisol messages – a phenomenon known as 'cortisol resistance'. In effect, these immune cells stop paying attention to cortisol and ignore its message to switch off inflammation.

Miller describes what is in effect a 'double whammy' for a child's health prospects: if early experiences are negative ones, the infant body may not only be desensitised to cortisol's messages, which makes it harder to turn off inflammation, but the immune system and its macrophages will also be programmed to react more strongly and to be *more* inflammatory than normal. As Greg Miller summed it up: 'As a consequence, persons exposed to early stress show chronic inflammation throughout life.' Miller and his colleagues have described this as like having a 'car that has a healthy accelerator and sluggish brakes'.[24]

This affects the individual's susceptibility to infection. In a small but significant study in 2012, Sheldon Cohen and his colleagues (including Gregory Miller) gathered some healthy volunteers. Some of them had been exposed to a recent major stressful experience associated with long-term threat, and had immune cells that had become relatively insensitive to cortisol (cortisol resistance) – although they were otherwise healthy. He went on to show how this affected their ability to deal with the cold virus. Exposing all his volunteers to a rhinovirus, he found the volunteers who were more likely to develop a cold were those who had cortisol resistance and were unable to control their inflammatory reactions.[25] In other words, it was not high cortisol itself but uncontrolled inflammation that was the health risk.

Many studies have demonstrated that maltreated children have more chronic inflammation: in particular, higher levels of the inflammatory cytokines IL-6 and CRP have been noted.[26] In fact, the pro-inflammatory cytokine IL-6 seems to be the cytokine of choice that the body releases in distressing, unsafe social relationships. Its release has been linked with a variety of unhappy early life experiences, such as hostility, anger, conflict, aggressive behaviour, physical abuse, as well as loneliness, depression and social isolation. At the other end of life, high levels of IL-6 have been associated with frailty and disability.[27]

This is notable as the chronic inflammatory state that begins in one's early years can become a permanent state of affairs and can be maintained through to adulthood. For example, one study looked at adults caring for relatives who had dementia. As might be expected, it was stressful being a carer, and indeed carers had higher levels of inflammatory IL-6 cytokines than other matched individuals in a control group. However, this only reached statistical significance in those carers who had also previously experienced abuse or adversity as children. As the distinguished psychologist Janice Kiecolt-Glaser and her team concluded of their study: 'Adverse childhood experiences have lasting, measurable consequences later in life, producing effects that were large enough to be perceptible beyond a major chronic stressor,

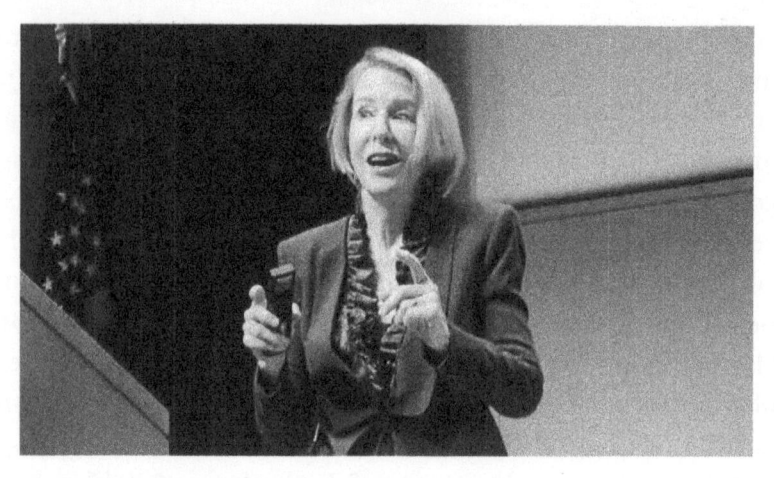

Professor Janice Kiecolt-Glaser, an American psychoneuroimmunologist who has explored the impact of stress on the immune and endocrine systems

dementia family caregiving [. . .] Childhood adversities cast a very long shadow.'[28]

What is inflammation for?

Acute inflammation is the body's urgent first defence against infection. Innate immune cells, such as neutrophils and macrophages, draw on omega-6 fatty acids to go on the offensive against infection. They release inflammatory cytokines to direct the fight-back, as well as powerful oxidants to destroy infection, followed up, if necessary, with a more targeted response to particular pathogens, from the adaptive immune system.

This short-term inflammation is often an effective defence. Problems arise only when inflammation is not resolved and gets out of control, when excessive prolonged presence of free radicals and oxidants can potentially damage normal cell structures, leading to disease[29] or when inflammation becomes chronic, such as in allergic responses and auto-immune (self-attacking) conditions.

Free radicals and oxidants are not only triggered by infection, but can also be generated by other assaults on bodily well-being, such as stress, pollution, smoking and alcohol, obesity, high blood sugar and early maltreatment. The healthy body then needs to rebalance by drawing on its antioxidant defences – the familiar positives, such as breastfeeding, exercise, and being in green spaces, as well as a healthy diet that includes vitamin E from nuts and grains, vitamin C from acid fruits, lycopene from tomatoes, and, indirectly, flavonoids from green tea, grapes, wine and chocolate – to restore a balance between the free radicals, oxidants and the antioxidants. However, when stress factors are too great, or the person's diet does not include enough fruit and vegetables to generate plentiful antioxidants, this process may fail and the balance tips in favour of oxidants, resulting in oxidative stress.

Oxidative stress creates risk for a variety of chronic and degenerative diseases, including cancer, diabetes, cardiovascular diseases and pulmonary disease, as well as some neurodegenerative conditions. Oxidative stress and inflammation usually go together and accentuate each other in a vicious cycle where oxidative stress triggers inflammation, which then stimulates the production of more oxidants. Inflammation plus oxidative stress are jointly involved in the pathogenesis of many diseases. So is the cure to take anti-oxidant supplements and to improve the diet? The biochemist Subrata Biswas reviewed these links and looked at attempts to treat illnesses such as diabetes, cardiovascular disease and cancer with antioxidant supplements. He found that trials of antioxidant supplements and diets were not that successful for people with cancer. As he explains it, anti-oxidants are good for maintaining health and *preventing* abnormal growths, but once a person already has malignant cancer cells, he or she will need oxidants to get rid of those cells.[30]

Calming inflammation

Although the battle against infection may demand harsh inflammatory and oxidant measures, it is vital that this process should come to a swift resolution. When inflammation cannot be resolved in a timely fashion, it turns into the problem, not the solution. Chronic inflammation, like chronic stress, can lead to more serious health damage.

The importance of resolving inflammation is increasingly coming into focus in scientific research as more is learnt about the process. While the classical understanding of an inflammatory response was that inflammation is a 'self-limiting' process – it just fades out when the original cause has been dealt with – new thinking suggests that the process of resolution demands a more active response from the macrophages. It now begins to look as if, rather than just fizzling out, inflammation ends when macrophages move into a second phase of activity.

The new version of events is that, at the peak of the acute inflammation, the macrophages start to prepare for inflammatory activity to wind down. To achieve this, they turn into a more mellow version of themselves. Drawing on omega-3 DHA fish oil (instead of omega-6), they start to make substances called specialised pro-resolving mediators (SPMs), which calm down the inflammatory process. They bring inflammation to a conclusion, partly by switching on the anti-inflammatory cytokine IL-10 and cortisol, bringing neutrophil activity to a halt. This second stage of macrophage activity is now focused on clearing up the dead neutrophils, and on releasing the soothing SPMs, allowing tissue healing to take place, particularly in the lining of the gut and the lining of the blood vessels.[31]

Without SPMs, unchecked inflammation can lead to destructive consequences. For example, some patients with uncontrolled lung inflammation, including clinically severe asthma, have a defect in the generation of specialised pro-resolving mediators.[32] Similarly, obesity also seems to create difficulty in resolving inflammation using SPMs. Recent work by Cristina López-Vicario and her colleagues suggests that this may be due to the diet of many obese people, which is characterised by an imbalance between omega-6 fatty acid and omega-3 fatty acid. When the diet is top-heavy with omega-6 foods, such as vegetable oils and soy oil found in processed foods, there may be more difficulty in generating pro-resolving mediators (SPMs) derived from omega-3.[33]

These discoveries are leading to a quest for new medication that takes account of this increased understanding of the way that inflammation is resolved. Past anti-inflammatory medications have primarily been targeted at reducing the symptoms of acute inflammation, such as swelling and pain. They have had some success in this role and are widely used (in fact, around 40% of older adults over sixty-five are thought to receive at least one prescription a year, many for drugs such as ibuprofen).

However, such drugs have not been particularly successful in resolving chronic inflammatory conditions. Used long-term, they can even have negative side effects, such as peptic ulcers.[34] It's also possible they may prevent macrophages from generating SPMs. Some scientists are now turning their attention to developing new treatments for chronic inflammation, such as the commercial production of 'resolvins' – one of the SPMs derived from omega-3 DHA. These might even have an impact on the devastating neuroinflammatory disorders such as Alzheimer's and Parkinson's diseases[35] – hopeful news for those of us who are caught in the trap of such conditions. However, it is not clear whether or not omega-3 DHA supplements would do the trick just as well; or whether manufactured resolvins are needed.[36]

Inflammation can be a killer

However, as already mentioned, inflammation is not only a reaction to infection or injury, but can also be triggered by a range of psychological stresses, from childhood maltreatment to social isolation to marital strife.

In particular, interpersonal stress has been linked to chronic inflammatory conditions such as rheumatoid arthritis, psoriasis, inflammatory bowel conditions and obesity.[37] Depression, too, is a common, disabling condition that has also been linked to psychological stress and high levels of inflammatory markers. One team of researchers described it as a 'pro-inflammatory state'.[38]

Some have speculated that it is pro-inflammatory cytokines that generate the familiar symptoms of depression – the 'sickness behaviour' many depressed people experience, such as lethargy, loss of appetite and inability to concentrate.[39] One new approach is to address this directly by treating depression with anti-inflammatories – a line of attack that is proving successful, according to a recent review of the clinical evidence from randomised controlled trials (RCTs) using anti-inflammatories either on their own or as 'add-ons' to other treatments.[40]

As well as initiating an inflammatory response, early stressful relationships, particularly emotional abuse, can also 'get into the belly', suppressing good bacteria in the gut and triggering 'bad' bacteria.[41] This unhealthy balance of gut bacteria has been linked to various diseases, including neurological diseases, chronic kidney diseases, type 2 diabetes and, increasingly, to cardiovascular diseases like atherosclerosis and stroke.[42] Microbes are even 'suspected to be involved in approximately 20% of cancers', according to Johan Gagniere and his colleagues in a global review for the World Journal of Gastroenterology.[43]

A poor diet may also play a key role, since poor eating practices, such as a lack of fibre in the diet, can lead to a less diverse microbiome. In particular, such diets may fail to generate enough of the SCFA (short chain fatty acid) butyrate, the substance that, among other things, protects the mucus barrier in the lining of the gut. A lack of butyrate has been linked to arterial stiffness[44] and to coronary artery disease.[45] Reduced numbers of butyrate-producing bacteria have also been found in patients with colon cancer, suggesting that a potential dietary influence on the mucus barrier might play a part in the condition.[46] New research also suggests that the health of the mucus barrier may also be important in neurological diseases such as Alzheimer's, Multiple Sclerosis and Parkinson's disease. All three conditions are characterised by constipation and all three are correlated with an increase of *Akkermansia muciniphila* bacteria.[47]

Together, unbalanced gut bacteria and chronic gut inflammation may become a key pathway to disease. Researcher Erica DeJong links the two together when she says '. . . virtually all chronic inflammatory conditions (e.g. cardiovascular disease, dementia and inflammatory disorders) are associated with microbial dysbiosis'.[48]

These outcomes become most obvious in old age, when the gut microbiota tends to change for the worse and when low grade chronic inflammation is more likely. Many of the most life-threatening conditions of older age are linked to chronic inflammation, often with their roots in early life.[49]

Some cancers fall into this category, since tissues damaged by inflammation are also more prone to develop cancers. For example, chronic acid reflux can contribute to the growth of tumours such as oesophageal cancer. These links may not be causal. However, the Northern Irish expert on ageing, Emeritus Professor Maeve Rea, is in no doubt that: 'many cancers arise from sites of infection, chronic irritation and inflammation'.[50]

Inflammation has even been implicated in the recent global coronavirus pandemic. Although infectious disease was, until recently, believed to be largely under control or vanquished in developed countries, coronavirus has proved the exception. The virus can lead to a dangerous 'cytokine storm' of lung inflammation in some patients, with some new evidence finding a correlation between those with low vitamin D and susceptibility to such uncontrollable inflammation.[51] Similarly, pre-existing chronic inflammation generated by obesity or diabetes may create a vulnerability to the virus and play a part in its high death toll. Heightened levels of inflammation can also lead to an unusual formation of blood clots or thromboses affecting many body systems simultaneously, which have also been implicated in some Covid-19 deaths.[52]

Dreadful and destructive as the coronavirus Covid-19 has been, it is not the greatest danger to life. Heart disease is still higher on the list of killers. More than 17 million deaths worldwide were attributed to cardiovascular disease in one year alone: 2016;[53] while Covid-19 accounts for approximately 7 or more million deaths worldwide in total at the time of writing.* Astonishingly large numbers of people in the USA have some form of cardiovascular disease – as many as 48%, if high blood pressure is included.[54] It is thought to kill one in three Americans. And, for many, it starts in childhood.

The route to cardiovascular disease

Atherosclerosis – a disease in which fatty plaques build up in the arteries – is thought to be the precursor of cardiovascular disease, and many scientists now believe that inflammation is at the heart of atherosclerosis. As the biochemist Amit Shrivastava put it, 'all stages of the atherosclerotic process, from its initiation to plaque rupture, might be considered an inflammatory response to injury and endothelial dysfunction'.[55]

The first step in cardiovascular disease and stroke is thought to be an inflamed 'endothelium', the inner lining of the blood vessels that carry blood around the body. A healthy smooth endothelium enables blood to flow well, keeping a balance between dilation and constriction of the arteries and veins and ensuring a stable blood pressure, as well as regulating blood clotting and managing inflammation. However, when the endothelium is damaged in some way,

---

* Latest WHO figures for January 2024 are of 7,010,681 deaths ('Covid 19 epidemiological update – 19 January 2024').

such as by oxidised LDL cholesterol particles, or when a blood clot forms and is not cleared away, other local substances can get caught up in the inflamed area and build up into plaque.

How is a healthy endothelium achieved? There is no great mystery: it flourishes with a healthy, active way of life and a good diet that does not contain too many sugars, and that includes antioxidants such as red wine and many plant-based foods. In particular, the endothelium is supported by those things that help blood flow freely to the body's organs – particularly physical exercise, which stimulates the release of nitric oxide from the endothelium. Perhaps more surprisingly, emotional well-being also plays a part. Positive social connections that generate oxytocin also stimulate nitric oxide.[56]

Conversely, a sedentary way of life, smoking and pollution has the opposite effect, reducing nitric oxide in the endothelium, constricting the blood vessels and increasing blood pressure as well as stiffening the arteries.[57] There are many sources of inflammation and oxidative stress that can trigger endothelial damage: the psychological stress of unhappy relationships, a lack of sleep, smoking or passive smoking, infections, and environmental pollution. Problems can start even in utero. A stressful pregnancy that leads to low birth weight can contribute to subsequent inflammation; this is thought to be a particular factor in racial disparities in cardiovascular health.[58] Equally, the mother being overweight or obese during pregnancy, which generates inflammatory cytokines from the visceral fat round her abdominal organs, can in turn affect the placenta, leading to endothelial cell dysfunction in the baby and increased risk of cardiovascular disease.[59]

Poor diet is particularly significant. Recent research has explored which unhealthy eating habits generate inflammation that can lead to endothelial dysfunction. A range of foods have been implicated. Top of the list is the impact of over-eating refined carbohydrates – such as white bread, white rice and white noodles – which have recently been identified as the single biggest food risk factor for cardiovascular disease.[60] Another route may be through the effect of fried and processed foods, which often contain excessive omega-6 vegetable oils (linoleic acid); this is a key factor in the oxidation of LDL (low density lipoprotein) cholesterol (popularly known as 'bad' cholesterol).[61] These are also the foods heavily marketed to and most popular with children.

One of the greatest dangers to health for young children, who cannot choose their lifestyles, is their extraordinary exposure to sugar. One expert, Robert Lustig, calculated that in our current food culture, 35% of children's calories come from sugar.[62] This is extremely risky, since endothelial cells are particularly sensitive to high levels of glucose.[63] An overload of glucose and fructose releases free radicals and leads to oxidative stress, which alters and damages the cells that line the blood vessels, making them 'bumpy'. This allows fatty particles, such as oxidised LDL, to stick to their surface.[64]

When oxidised LDL cholesterol particles get embedded in the artery wall, they raise a red flag to the immune system. The white blood cells – macrophages – are alerted to potential trouble and come to fix the damage. As they eat up the fatty LDL cholesterol, they become foam cells, which turn into fatty streaks. This can begin in early life, often in childhood, and in some cases in the womb. Some babies are even born with fatty streaks in their coronary arteries. This unhealthy start in life is associated with some of the usual suspects, particularly with parents' smoking and raised LDL cholesterol levels.[65] There are also some genetic hyper-lipidaemia conditions.

Slowly, these streaks accumulate and contribute to forming plaques – which are essentially pools of fat surrounded by a build-up of local debris, such as calcified material and fibrous tissue – with a thin crust around the edge.

Gradually, plaques merge, thickening the lining of the blood vessel and blocking the free flow of blood until some further stress

Unprotected: stressful relationships and how they affect health

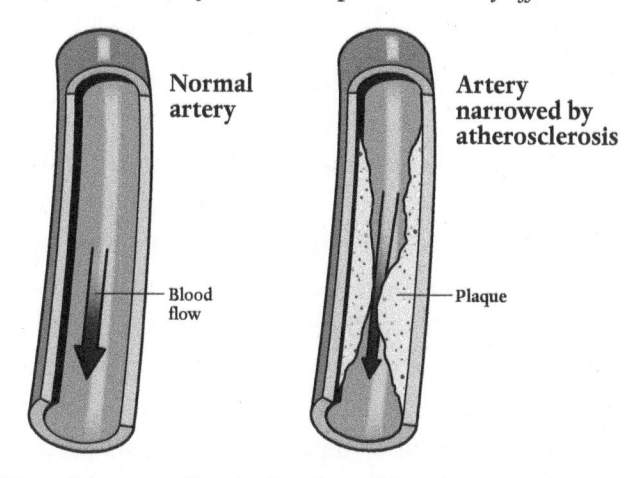

How plaque can affect the free flow of blood through the artery

triggers a rupture.[66] Some moment of intensified stress – whether from a surge in heart rate and blood pressure due to intense physical exertion or a psychological challenge, or due to infection and inflammation – leads to cracking or rupturing of the thin cap around the plaque. Necrotic (dead) cells and plaque material ooze out, potentially blocking the artery or triggering the formation of blood clots that can block the artery.

One of the earliest warning signs for atherosclerosis is a thickening of the lining of the arteries. Known as 'intima media thickness', this is regarded as a 'preclinical' marker of atherosclerosis, and it can start very young, even in the womb. Building on David Barker's seminal work on poor nutrition in pregnancy and its links to heart disease, more recent work confirms that a mother's undernutrition in pregnancy – such as a lack of calories or a lack of protein in her diet in early pregnancy – can increase the risk of her child developing a thickening of the lining of the blood vessels by the time he or she is nine years old.[67] Similarly, children who are obese are also more likely to have increased thickening of the lining of the arteries after the age of nine, and for this to continue into adulthood.[68]

When chickens come home to roost

Such invisible processes at the start of life may unknowingly set the child up for ill health in later life, a long journey that can end in cardiovascular disease many years later.[69] As we age, the metaphorical chickens come home to roost. Cardiovascular risk increases as we age. Ageing decreases elastin fibres in the arterial wall, hardening it, particularly if there is not enough 'good' HDL cholesterol to help keep the arteries soft.[70] As the body starts to wear out, inflammation can become more difficult to manage and resolve, partly because there can be a loss of SPMs (specialised pro-resolving mediators), as well as decreased oxytocin levels, which normally would have an anti-inflammatory role as well as playing a part in regulating blood pressure and reducing heart rate. As we age, there is also increased oxidative stress (too many oxidants, not enough anti-oxidants to counter them).

In the deeply unfair luck of the draw, those who suffered most in childhood are more likely to face poor health in later life. In fact, early life stress is a 'robust predictor' of risk for cardiovascular disease and stroke.[71] Childhood sexual abuse, in particular, has been associated with intima media thickening of the arteries in middle age.[72] As we've already covered, three or more adverse childhood experiences (ACEs) are also linked with increased risk of heart disease.[73] This risk is particularly great for those ageing adults who had to deal with social and psychological stress in childhood and developed a heightened reactivity to stress with high levels of cortisol. Such prolonged exposure to cortisol over the years is associated with severe and progressively increasing calcification of the coronary artery over time.[74]

This is significant because the degree of coronary artery calcification is increasingly being seen as the most accurate way to predict cardiovascular risk. Relatively straightforward scans for coronary artery calcification (CAC scores) are thought by some likely to become the cardiovascular equivalent of regular mammograms for breast cancer. Such tests indirectly reveal the state of the arteries. Since calcium is attracted to the fatty plaques, the very presence of calcium suggests there is plaque in the arteries. Those lucky enough to have a zero coronary artery calcification score are in effect being given something like a '15-year warranty against heart attack'.[75]

These lucky owners of such a desirable 'warranty' are likely to be those who have enjoyed the positive relationships, particularly in early life, that kept inflammation at bay. This was corroborated by a longitudinal study undertaken at the University of Turku in Finland, which showed an independent association between childhood psychosocial well-being and reduced coronary artery calcification in adulthood.[76] Perhaps, one day, CAC scans might be part of a routine package of preventive measures for people identified as sufferers of ACEs in childhood.

Cancer's roots in early life

The impact of early stress on the risk of other major diseases, such as cancer, is less clear. This is partly because cancer develops in stages over a lengthy period of time and often involves multiple causes. With that said, there are studies that show a possible link between childhood experiences and later cancer development. One study in particular looked at a large cohort of European Jews who emigrated to Israel. A study of the later health of these émigrées found that they had high incidence rates of all cancers. However, the largest effects were seen in those people who had been born during 1940–1945, who had been exposed to the dangers and terrors of the Holocaust as very young children, before the age of five. Compared to émigrées of the same generation who arrived in Israel before the war, the children who were born under Nazi rule before emigrating had a much higher risk for all cancers (elevated 3.5-fold).[77]

There are many suggestive links between unhappy or traumatic early experiences and later cancer. For example, Michelle Kelly-Irving and her colleagues at the University of Toulouse in France found that two or more adverse childhood experiences (ACEs) doubled women's risk of having a cancer before the age of fifty.[78] However, it is difficult to prove that stress directly *causes* cancer. A recent study of people with incurable chronic lymphocytic leukaemia could only say that psychological stress was related to heightened levels of the inflammatory cytokine markers that are associated with progressive disease.[79] Others have suggested that up to a quarter of all cancers arise 'in association with' chronic inflammation. Inflammation has been linked with particular cancers, such as colorectal cancer, as well as those of the uterus, liver, bladder, oesophagus and stomach.

One way of explaining how an inflammatory environment may be linked to cancer is that a grumbling inflammatory condition can lead to the production of excessive oxidants. If unchecked by antioxidants, this can hinder normal processes, such as the clearing away of dead infected cells (apoptosis), and can cause mutations in tumour suppressor genes that normally keep abnormal growths in check.[80] Chronic inflammation can cause tissue damage, which creates an environment predisposed to new abnormal growth.[81] If pro-inflammatory cytokines continue to be released, they can then 'influence tumour promotion, survival, proliferation, invasion, angiogenesis and metastases'.[82]

Difficult relationships deprive children of a cushion against stress

It's tempting to focus attention exclusively on the health impact of negative experiences. But it's equally important to recognise the importance of good relationships in protecting our health.

Stress is an inevitable part of life. A certain amount of stress is needed to get up in the morning, to keep us active, productive and positive. Mild stress can even act as a kind of inoculation against more severe stress.[83] Problems arise when stress becomes overwhelming and stops the individual from functioning. This is not just due to the quantity or intensity of the stressful experience itself, but also depends on the individual's endowment of stress responsiveness and ability to manage stress. A healthy person is one who has had good enough early nutrition to ensure bodily systems function well and good enough early relationships to have confidence that others will help to manage their stress when necessary. Reliable, secure relationships are essential for body and mind to flourish and make it possible to regulate emotions, and to keep stress and inflammation in check. They not only provide a psychological buffer, but also aid physiological recovery processes.

When these conditions are not met in early life, the child's vulnerability to disease increases. One intriguing study, based on a large sample of Harvard students in the 1950s, followed them up in middle age. It found that those who had described their childhood relationship with their mothers and fathers as 'warm' and 'close' had better health in later life. Those who didn't experience such warmth were twice as likely to have conditions such as coronary artery disease, hypertension, duodenal ulcers and alcoholism.[84]

How do loving relationships protect health? One part of the answer, at least, is that warm, connected families are more likely to provide effective ways of managing and recovering from stress and inflammation. According to one large, recent Canadian study of children and teenagers, the relationship between lack of social support and inflammation emerges early in life. Feeling connected to a social network and feeling valued by others has been found to lower IL-6.[85] In insecure families, on the other hand, many of the body's defensive reactions can become chronically activated, particularly the inflammatory response and the stress response. As previously described, chronic stress can leave the HPA axis stress response dysregulated – either blunted or hyper-reactive – allowing the immune system to develop a pro-inflammatory phenotype, and disturbing the health of the gut microbiome. There are clear links between insecure attachment relationships in the first year of life and the likelihood of developing chronic inflammation-based illnesses in adulthood, according to one long-term prospective study by neuropsychologist Jennifer Puig and her colleagues at the University of Minnesota.[86] These findings were echoed by a smaller, more recent study, which also found that poor quality early relationships in the first months of life had a stronger influence over future functioning than more obvious adversities, such as poverty.[87] Equally importantly, the protective soothing systems established in early life may also become less effective.

The balm of oxytocin

The contribution that warm relationships make to health is most clearly seen in the case of the hormone oxytocin. As described earlier in Chapter 5, oxytocin is generated by safe and enjoyable physical closeness and touch and by feeling cared for.

Oxytocin also 'plays a pivotal role in the development and functions of the immune system'.[88] There are receptors for oxytocin in immune cells and organs. Oxytocin has a direct impact on health because it promotes development of the thymus gland, which generates the T-cells that kill off infections. However, it has other healing functions, such as moderating or even suppressing inflammatory cytokines. It can also inhibit HPA axis activation and can slow down or suppress the release of cortisol. It facilitates wound healing, and may also stimulate repair and survival of the heart muscle cells, alleviating cardiovascular problems.[89] Oxytocin is like a protective balm that almost seems to have been designed to counteract the impact of stress on the body.

However, children who experience the benefits of oxytocin are living in a different world from those whose infant relationships have been marred by neglectful, insensitive or abusive parenting.

Unprotected: stressful relationships and how they affect health

For them, this buffer against stress and inflammation is not available. Evidence suggests that children neglected in orphanages, those who experience early separations from their attachment figure or who live with stressful or insecure attachment relationships between parents and child, all generate less oxytocin.[90] Some research suggests that genetic factors may also be at play, as some children with genes for high oxytocin receptor expression are more sensitive to a negative social environment. Those who are mistreated as children are then at greater risk that their own parenting, in turn, will be more negative.[91]

In these negative situations, oxytocin receptor genes are more likely to be switched off or 'methylated' (as are their glucocorticoid receptors), and we are more likely to grow up with anxiety, depression and distrust of others. Instead of socially flourishing, we become less capable of enjoying close relationships.[92]

Can you make up for lost oxytocin?

Recently, two experts on oxytocin, Ben Buemann and Kerstin Uvnas-Moberg, undertook a review of the potential future use of oxytocin as a therapy, particularly as a protection against heart disease. It looked promising, as it had become possible to administer oxytocin by nasal spray. One commercial company even offered it for sale as a spray marketed as 'Liquid Trust' – claiming to enhance social confidence and empathy in the wearer.

However, research projects to explore its effects when delivered in this form have had mixed results. Oxytocin sprays worked for stressed baby rats separated from their mothers,[93] and some studies also had positive results with autistic children, but these were convincing with younger children only.[94] Other studies found that giving an oxytocin nasal spray to those who had experienced early adversities and unsupportive parenting did not show any improvement in social behaviour and, in some cases, even had a negative response to the administration of oxytocin later on.[95] Rather than use a spray, Buemann and Uvnas-Moberg would prefer us to enhance oxytocin by natural means, by supporting 'more and better social bonds'. However, they acknowledge that this is difficult to pursue through the health services. Living up to the Scandinavian stereotype, instead they conclude that it might be easier for medical professionals to recommend frequent exercise and sexual and tactile pleasures.[96]

Many decades ago, Felitti and Anda alerted us to the impact of childhood stress and its effects on lifelong health, breaking the taboo on linking emotions and physical health that had prevailed since Enlightenment thinkers separated mind and body. They asked a radical new question, 'What happened to you?', which was the key to understanding so much more about the influence of early experience on developing physiological systems. Today the biological processes that are involved are getting ever clearer, but there is still much to discover. As Felitti and Anda first highlighted, it is now undisputed that chronically stressful childhood experiences have wide-ranging physiological consequences for adult health. At the same time, we know that the immune system and other whole-body systems flourish in conditions of safety and well-being. Inevitably, this raises important questions about our social priorities and how we might ensure those conditions for all children – both inside the family, but also outside it.

7
Child poverty and health

> 'Poverty is about more than money . . . Poverty is more like a gravitational field comprising social, economic, emotional, physiological, political and cultural forces.'
>
> Darren McGarvey, 2017

> 'Poverty is neither simply an act of God nor something people do, or don't do, to themselves. The level of child poverty in a society is under a great deal of political control. It is a choice made by the political system.'
>
> Michael Marmot, *The Health Gap*

Although families have a powerful influence on children, wider contexts also matter to our health. This is most obvious when considering the poorest one billion people, suffering from extreme poverty and struggling to survive. Many live in rural sub-Saharan Africa or South Asia, where life expectancy is short due to the huge challenge to get enough to eat, to have safe drinking water, to breathe clean air or to be protected from unsafe roads. In these perilous environments, death from drowning, road injuries and asthma are major risks, as well as the continuing threat of infectious disease.[1] However, even in the most privileged Western societies, people in the poorest groups still have a greatly increased risk of disease and shorter lives. What are the key factors that lead to these outcomes?

The epidemiologist Michael Marmot, renowned for his explorations of the relationship between income and health, says that what links poverty in different countries, even though the concept of 'poverty' is set at very different levels of income, is a shared loss of 'opportunity, empowerment and security'. In other words, poverty is not just about the physical experience of lack of health care or food, it is also a psychosocial experience connected to an individual's relationship to others. When this relationship reflects an imbalance of power and conveys a lack of care, stress and ill health may result.

The stress associated with relative poverty and low socio-economic status has some similar but subtly different characteristics to the stress explored in the previous chapter. Above all, it is characterised by an experience of lack of control, as well as feelings of devaluation – this time by the wider social group rather than by individuals within the family. Experiences of inequality, such as racism and discrimination, exclusion, being paid wages that are inadequate to live on, having little choice of housing, can all contribute to this feeling of lack of worth.

As Darren McGarvey describes, in his book *Poverty Safari*, the stress of poverty is 'all-consuming: it's the soup everyone is swimming in all the time'.[2] Without resources, many needs simply can't be met, and there is no cushion or margin for error. One American, who grew up to become a wealthy Wall Street trader after a poor and hungry childhood, described the key feature of being poor as a lack of control over events – for example, if your phone is cut off because you can't pay the bill, you may lose a job you are trying to get. As he put it: 'The reality is that when you're poor, if you make one mistake, you're done'.[3] A similar sense of precarity was expressed by Jack Monroe, a British food blogger, who gave evidence to the UK parliament of her experience of poverty. Lacking cash to pay even a small bill can lead to escalating problems – 'how quickly a £6 water charge can spiral into hundreds of pounds in late fees and bank charges, and nobody will give you the smallest of overdrafts, to tide you over . . .'[4]

Part of the stress of poverty comes from a sense that you and your feelings are of little importance to the wider society. As Linda Tirado, a woman surviving on two minimum wage jobs, described it, she dared not complain about her unpleasant conditions of work or home life, fearing a judgemental response – what she called 'The Look' –from professionals such as doctors and social workers. She defiantly spits out: 'Maybe feelings are something that only professional people have. My friends and I know that no one gives a shit about ours.'[5] Similarly, after the riots in London and other British cities in 2011, some of the young rioters reported feeling that 'no one cares about us'. One sixteen-year-old, Omar, who lacked qualifications and could not find a job, said he stole Nike tracksuit bottoms to make him feel like the 'people with money, good families', whom he felt looked down on him. 'I hate feeling people are judging me. They don't know about me and then they just look at you and I hate it, I absolutely hate it.'[6] Black people targeted for 'Stop and Search' by the police have described similar feelings of humiliation; former professional footballer Paul Mortimer described how, when it happened to him, 'people walk by and look and perceive you to be a certain way. You never forget those types of looks

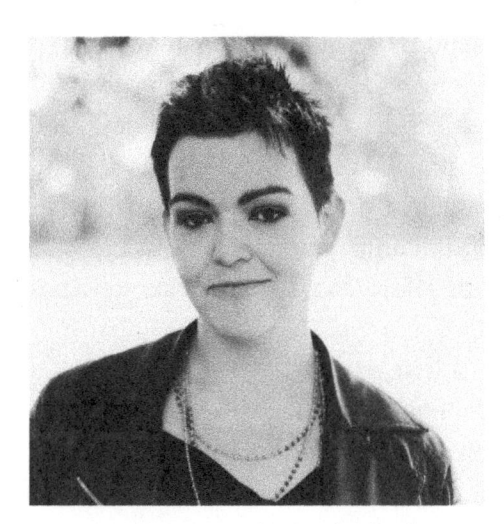

American journalist Linda Tirado

from people. The impact it had on me was huge, huge . . . I felt that I needed a shower after.'[7]

Anger and frustration are one response. Tirado herself cherished her anger, which sustained her energy. As she put it, it could 'punch through the haze' of depression at not being valued. Others collapse into hopelessness and helplessness. Depression is particularly prevalent in low-income mothers of young children, many of whom are single parents.

Living at the bottom of the social heap can generate feelings of rage and helplessness, which are intensely stressful emotions. The lack of control often extends to the physical environment too. Those with fewest resources have least choice and are more likely to live in less desirable areas of air pollution near major roads or under the flight paths of airplanes, furthest away from green spaces. Housing is more likely to be temporary, damp or overcrowded, situated in neighbourhoods full of other stressed individuals, some of whom may at times lose control of themselves and erupt in violence or vandalism.

To add insult to injury, the individualistic ideology of our current society blames the poor for their own poverty. As David Gordon's tongue-in-cheek alternative 'top 10 tips for health' parodies:

1. 'Don't be poor. If you can, stop. If you can't, try not to be poor for long.
2. Don't live in a deprived area. If you do, move.
3. Don't be disabled or have a disabled child.
4. Don't work in a stressful, low-paid manual job.
5. Don't live in damp, low-quality housing or be homeless.
6. Be able to afford to pay for social activities and annual holidays.
7. Don't be a lone parent.
8. Claim all benefits to which you are entitled.
9. Be able to afford to own a car.
10. Use education to improve your socio-economic position.'[8]

The body reacts to living in a harsh, unempathic society in much the same way that it reacts to harsh or neglectful parenting. It is on high alert to threat. The stress response may be chronically activated, and the immune system may also produce chronic inflammation. This may have its strongest impact in the first two years of life, as stress at this early stage of development can lead to a permanently heightened inflammatory response to stress, with lifelong health consequences.[9]

However, what matters most is how it feels to the person concerned. Not everyone experiences low socio-economic status in the same way. But researchers are increasingly homing in on one key factor that has a particularly negative impact on health – the feeling of not being in control.[10] Those individuals who started life in low socio-economic circumstances, but as adults have gained a sense of control over their life, have better health outcomes and longevity.[11] Similarly, when those of low socio-economic status report feeling satisfied with their lives, their stress hormone (cortisol) levels are much the same as those of high socio-economic circumstances individuals.[12]

Social support, or the lack of it, can also change the subjective experience of stress. When people feel connected to others who they can trust, with whom they can make plans, they are buffered to some degree from stress. As the late comedian Robin Williams quipped, quoting a line from one of his movies: 'I used to think the worst thing in life was to end up all alone. It's not. The worst thing in life is to end up with people who make you feel all alone.'[13] The feeling of isolation has a negative effect on the body. A consistent finding is that pregnant women with 'diminished social networks', who feel unsupported towards the end of their pregnancy, have higher levels of c-reactive protein (CRP), a key indicator of inflammation.[14]

On the other hand, positive experiences of social support or the support of a partner, have remarkable powers to promote positive physiological effects: it can lower blood pressure, reduce the stress hormone cortisol and lower pro-inflammatory cytokines, as well as increasing oxytocin and stimulating the activity of immune 'natural killer' cells that are involved in killing tumour cells and viruses.[15] In fact, the increased oxytocin generated by warm human interaction itself reduces HPA axis stress activity.[16] In infancy, children from low socio-economic backgrounds are protected from stressful experiences and an over-reactive inflammatory response if they have someone supportive with them to help them cope.[17]

Stressed parents and their health habits

However, when human relationships don't work well, most people across the social spectrum will reach for other ways to de-stress and find comfort. The most readily available, immediate methods tend to be smoking, drinking alcohol, taking drugs or eating sugary and fatty food. Although these coping mechanisms are used widely across society, those who rely most heavily on them can find themselves caught in addictive patterns that change brain physiology. Often these habits are formed before we fully realise how they might compromise our future health – or how they might have strong unwanted effects on our children, most strikingly during pregnancy when mother and offspring share her body.

Shared smoking

Smoking during pregnancy, for example, is most common in deprived populations, and especially among younger mothers. Averaged out over the whole country, the rate of smoking during pregnancy is around 10% of mothers – but in economically deprived areas, this rises dramatically. In the northern holiday resort of Blackpool, one of the most disadvantaged areas of Britain, 27% of pregnant women smoke.

Child poverty and health

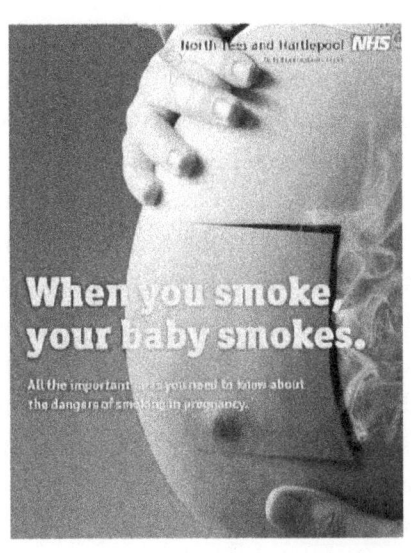

Poster from the 2017 NHS campaign against smoking in pregnancy

The children of smokers pay a high price. They are exposed to substances that irritate and damage a range of developing organs and body systems. One effect of smoking is that it raises the mother's baseline cortisol levels, which may then be passed on in the womb to her fetus, affecting its sensitivity to stress.[18] Another possible consequence is that maternal smoking can reduce lung function in the baby, and increase the child's risk for respiratory diseases.[19]

Smoking can also impair the baby's growth, including growth of the baby's higher brain areas, responsible for emotional self-control, potentially increasing the risk of hyperactivity and conduct disorders.[20] Most immediately problematic, though, is that maternal smoking is strongly linked to many cases of stillbirth or cot death.

Fast sugar

Even more common than smoking, sugar – in the form of sugar-laden soft drinks, or fast-release white carbohydrates – has become a socially acceptable way of alleviating stress. Growing evidence suggests that sugar can turn off the HPA stress response and lower levels of the stress hormone cortisol.[21] Sugar has also been shown to activate the release of oxytocin, which can also reduce HPA activity.[22]

The stress-busting qualities of sugar were demonstrated by one unusual study that followed young teenagers living in low-income neighbourhoods for a month. It supplied them with mobile phones that bleeped twice a day, asking them to record whether they had seen any physical fights at home or elsewhere that day. It also asked them to record their intake of vegetables, and to note whether they had eaten any fast food or drunk any fizzy or caffeinated drinks that day. The study clearly showed that, on days when the teenagers were exposed to violence, they consumed more fizzy and caffeinated drinks.[23]

Perhaps we should not be surprised, then, that people on or below the US poverty line (who are most exposed to violence) spend a whopping 9% of their income on soft drinks.[24] Sugar is cheap and readily available. It not only alleviates distress but also triggers the release of serotonin and a pleasurable surge of dopamine in the brain, just as alcohol and other drugs such as cocaine do.

This means that sugar, too, can become addictive. As with other addictions, consuming sugar can become compulsive and unrelated to appetite. As the drug abuse expert Nora Volkow has described the process of addiction, the brain gradually adapts to heavy consumption of sugar/alcohol/cocaine by shutting down dopamine receptors. This reduces the feelings of pleasure and reward generated by dopamine, so the individual has to increase consumption to ever higher levels to feel good. Once addicted, less dopamine is available to the brain, particularly in the areas of the brain involved in self-control and managing behaviour.[25]

This overconsumption of sugar – whether from fast processed food, sweets, carbs or alcohol – can become a way of life and, in time, lead to being overweight or obesity. This is one of the key factors in the obesity epidemic. However, although obesity affects all sections of society, in high-income Western nations, the risk of obesity is greatest for children born into poverty. Children who live in poverty or social disadvantage are more likely to have a higher BMI, and have a 20% higher risk of obesity in adulthood than those not in poverty.[26] In England's most deprived areas (defined by the government as areas suffering a combination of lower incomes, fewer jobs, less available housing, worse local environments, more crime, and worse health), 40% of children were overweight or obese in 2016, according to the Royal College of Paediatrics and Child Health.[27] This relationship between social class and body mass index (BMI) can even appear as early as the first year of life.

There are links between a mother's high consumption of sugar during pregnancy and the likelihood of her fetus becoming an overweight child. High intake of sugary drinks in mid-pregnancy, in particular, is associated with a child being overweight by school age.[28] Similar findings suggest that weight *gain* in early pregnancy also increases the chances of the fetus becoming overweight by the ages of six to nine years old,[29] with all its associated health risks. One way this may work is that a mother's over-consumption of sugar in pregnancy can increase the number of fat cells in the fetus – a state of affairs that sets up a lifelong capacity to lay down more fat.[30]

Another route is that the overweight or obese mother has unhealthy gut bacteria characteristic of obesity (such as bacteroides fragilis), which she may pass on to her infant either in the womb or through breastmilk. One prospective study found that the state of our microbiome aged two is highly predictive of our BMI aged twelve[31] – opening up the possibility of screening children's microbiomes and intervening early to protect a person from being overweight or obese in the future.

The link between a mother's obesity and her child's weight is a complex issue, which is hard to summarise. It is easy to fall into the trap of targeting (and blaming) individual health habits as the cause of obesity. However, this is not the full picture. As the delightfully named epidemiologist Summer Hawkins and her colleagues put it, we need to try to hold in mind the combination of social 'above-water' factors, such as political policies, neighbourhoods and families, that interact with biological 'underwater' factors, such as genes, epigenetics and physiology.[32] These bigger-picture issues are not under individual control, yet can influence our long-term physical health.

Certainly the stress of living with fewer resources can trigger unhealthy health choices. Mothers who consume a lot of sugar during pregnancy tend to be from the same demographic as those who smoke during pregnancy: young, low socio-economic status, poorly educated and overweight. In the post-natal period, these are also the mothers who are less likely to breastfeed, another factor that contributes to childhood obesity risk, as formula-fed babies are more likely to be obese.[33] One factor that contributes to this is the expectation, when bottle-feeding, that the baby should finish her bottle before stopping, rather than following her own body signals. Breast-fed babies, on the other hand, are better able to regulate their own intake, seeking milk when they are hungry and stopping their feed when they are full. In effect, the bottle-fed baby gets fewer meals, which are much bigger, and can more easily end up overfed. Despite this, Western culture has embraced formula milk. It is used by most parents in the first six months. This contributes to the rising levels of child obesity. Research increasingly suggests that formula-fed babies become heavier toddlers, are two and a half times more likely to be obese by age two, and by the age of six years old have a 12% increased risk of obesity.[34] Breastfeeding has been devalued in many low socio-economic-status communities – even associated with shame and revulsion. As one woman explained: 'If I breastfeed in Starbucks the whole café's just gonna leave.'[35] Women living in the most deprived areas are the least likely to breastfeed their babies. In relatively affluent Brighton and Hove, for example, figures from 2016/17 showed that 69% of babies were still being breastfed totally or partially by the time of their six-to-eight-week check-up, while in Blackpool the figure was only 25%. As Blackpool Council described it, 'the dominant culture within the town is one of bottle feeding'.[36]

Some of these bottle-feeding mothers will be single parents, perhaps feeling the pressure to return quickly to work. Other mothers may be influenced by cultural factors. Some people's reasons for turning away from breastfeeding can be surprising. In one US study, some women of colour from deprived backgrounds described wanting their baby 'to be strong and independent', believing that breastfeeding might lead to the baby being 'lazy' or 'spoiled' and less able to survive in a tough neighbourhood.[37] African-American attitudes in particular may also be shaped by history. This study also suggests that such communities may choose formula milk in part as a reaction to their ancestral experience of 'forced wet-nursing during slavery' or as a response to a past 'inability to purchase expensive breastmilk substitutes during the rise of "scientific motherhood" in the 1950s and 1960s', when formula milk first became popular.[38] However, the evidence appears to be different in the UK, where studies suggest that black and ethnic minority mothers have a slightly higher rate of breastfeeding.

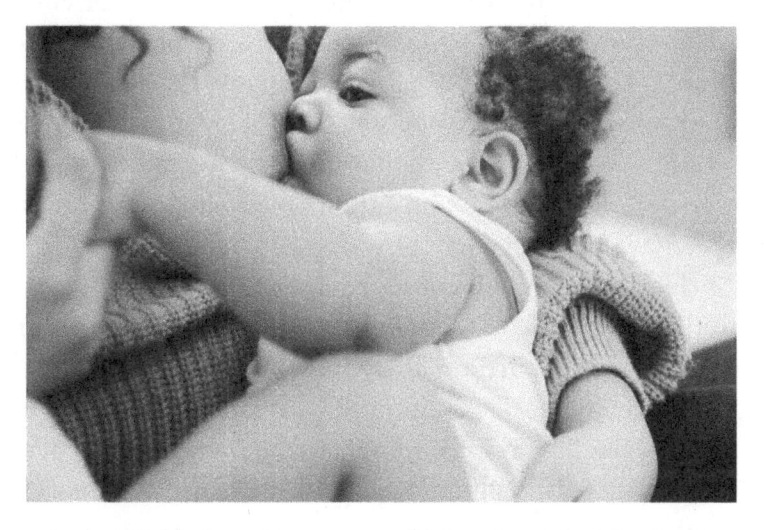

In the UK, black mothers are more likely to breastfeed, but in the US, they are least likely

In my work with parents and babies over a period of many years, I have encountered many reasons why disadvantaged families might choose not to breastfeed. On a practical level, breastfeeding is highly time-consuming. This can pose particular difficulties for poorer single mothers single-handedly caring for more than one child. Even when a disadvantaged mother does have a partner, he or she may not be supportive of breastfeeding, due to the stresses of his or her own life, such as long working hours. Some may feel jealous of their baby's privileged access to the mother's body and attention, or resentment at the sleep deprivation that feeding on demand may involve. These real pressures on the mother mean that, without strong support from other family or community members, breastfeeding is unlikely to succeed, as new mothers may not feel sufficiently motivated to persist and overcome its potential early difficulties.

Post-natal diet

Young children share the lives of their parents and their culture, including their dietary habits, which in turn are shaped by the food industry. A British survey of 2,477 low-income households found that the poorest families are not only more likely to drink more soft drinks and to eat more sugar and processed food, but are also less likely to eat vegetables or wholegrain breads. It seems unrealistic to expect families to change their eating patterns when they have young children. The evidence suggests that they don't. In fact, for children in the low-income families surveyed, the average consumption of veg was 1.6 portions a day (boys) or 2 portions (girls) – a long way from 'Five a day'.[39] According to most recent figures from the NHS Health Survey for England, average consumption of fruit and vegetables for all children aged five to fifteen was more like three a day.[40]

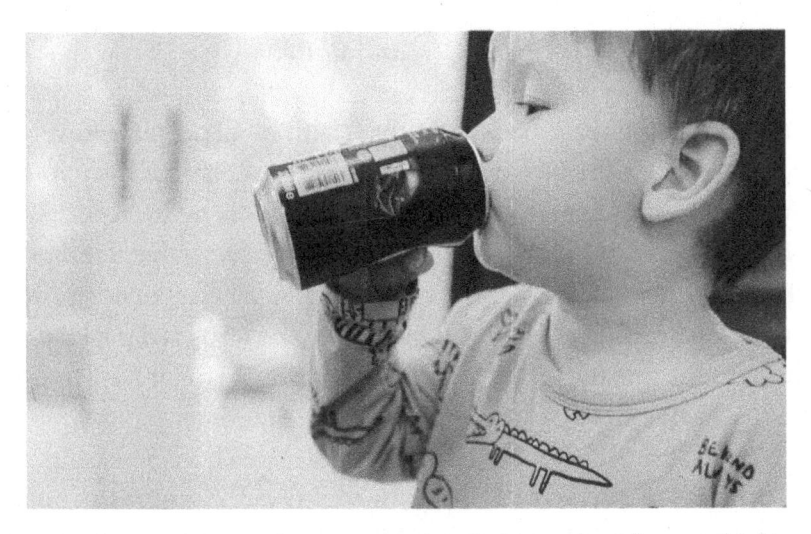

Despite the growing use of sugar taxes, many babies and toddlers are drinking sugar-sweetened drinks

In a food culture where it is commonplace to consume sugary and caffeinated drinks, it is perhaps inevitable that these will be offered even to very young children. Again, this is more prevalent in low-income families, even more so where mothers are depressed, or single-parent households, and also not breastfeeding. In their fascinating US study, anthropologists Amanda Thompson and Margaret Bentley made the extraordinary discovery that 78% of three-month-old babies in their low-income sample received age-inappropriate solid foods, including 20% who were already being given foods such as chips, crisps, maple syrup and ice cream, as well as fruit juice.[41] But these feeding practices are a direct line to future obesity. High consumption of sugary drinks and carbs in the first six months of life, as well as being given solid food before the age of four months, both strongly increase the odds of being diagnosed obese by the age of three. High consumption of sugary drinks at a year old has also been linked to cardio-metabolic risk in boys of school age.[42]

Obesity – and illness

Obesity in childhood matters for the health of all people. However, it has become a key factor in undermining the health of the poorest in society. Although any obese child is more likely to become an obese adult, with all the health risks associated with that condition, child obesity rates don't affect all children equally. As obesity levels have risen dramatically across society since the 1980s, it has increased faster in the most deprived communities, where 13% of four-to-five-year-olds are obese.[43]

The health risks of obesity are serious. As well as increasing the risks of heart disease and cancer in adulthood, obesity is strongly linked to type 2 diabetes – a condition that has been spiralling out of control, quadrupling since around 1980, to around 300 million patients worldwide, and which is disproportionately experienced by the most deprived.

Once again, it is important to note that early experiences matter. Type 2 diabetes is a disease that develops for many years before diagnosis. It may seem surprising that warning signs can be seen as early as at aged eight years old; a large study found that children who have lower levels of HDL ('good') cholesterol at this age, and increased markers of inflammation, are already at greater risk of chronic diabetic illness as middle-aged adults.[44]

All the usual culprits are implicated in setting up the conditions for diabetes type 2: in particular, those practices that contribute to inflammation and oxidative stress. These include smoking and lack of exercise, but also stress, such as childhood neglect or abuse in early life (such maltreatment is linked to later low levels of HDL 'good' cholesterol). However, diet is usually seen as the number-one factor, and is most implicated in 'sweet blood'. Diets overly full of glucose can lead to insulin resistance, where insulin becomes ineffective in managing glucose. The insulin receptor on the cell surface no longer lets glucose in, leaving high levels circulating in the blood, which can lead to inflammation of the lining of the blood vessels.

As previously described, inflammation may also result from eating the kind of diet full of cheap processed foods that has too much omega-6 relative to omega-3 fatty acids. Similarly, too much high-fructose corn syrup stimulates inflammation and leads to unhealthy bacteria in the gut.[45] To make matters worse, such diets often lack fibrous vegetables, which can lead to a lack of the beneficial short-chain fatty acids (SCFAs) and their protective, anti-inflammatory effect.

Politics of food

Many commentators are no longer pulling their punches about the significance of food practices in creating ill health. The food writer Bee Wilson put it starkly: 'our food is killing us',[46] while the prestigious medical journal *The Lancet* also stated its view that diet was 'the leading cause of poor health globally'.[47] Conflicts around the politics of food are escalating as it becomes clear that politicians have failed to regulate the food industry and have avoided long-term thinking about how to achieve a sustainable food system as the planet overheats. In the absence of a plan, the likelihood is that, in the near future, agriculture will start to produce lower yields, the nutrient content of food will be reduced, and we will face recurrent food crises.

Again the ideology of individualism would prefer to attribute responsibility to the individual consumer, who is portrayed as having a free choice over their diet. If only the poorest people in society would stop eating cheap fast food, ready meals and sugary snacks! If only they would stop living in run-down estates and neighbourhoods where the local shop or supermarket has little fresh produce or charges a premium price for fruit and vegetables!

It is wrong to blame individuals for decisions made by manufacturers. It is food producers (with government collusion) who choose to lace so much food with emulsifiers, preservatives, artificial food colours – many linked with allergies, hyperactivity, damage to the gut mucus, and endocrine disruption.[48] Individuals are also not responsible for government decisions to subsidise production of corn syrup so that it becomes cheap enough to use in everything from soft drinks to bread to yoghurt to ketchup and fruit juice, creating a silent mass addiction to sugar of which most consumers are unaware.

It is no coincidence that both the obesity epidemic and the diabetes epidemic have soared since the early 1980s, when the US government introduced substantial subsidies for certain crops, such as corn and grains, diverting farming away from crops with less predictable yields, such as fruit and vegetable production. Half the agricultural land in the USA now grows corn and soy. As a result of so much corn becoming available, the ultra-sweet high-fructose corn syrup became the cheap alternative to sugar and its consumption rose from virtually zero in 1970 to over 60 pounds a year per person by the year 2000,[49] particularly in the form of sweetened beverages.

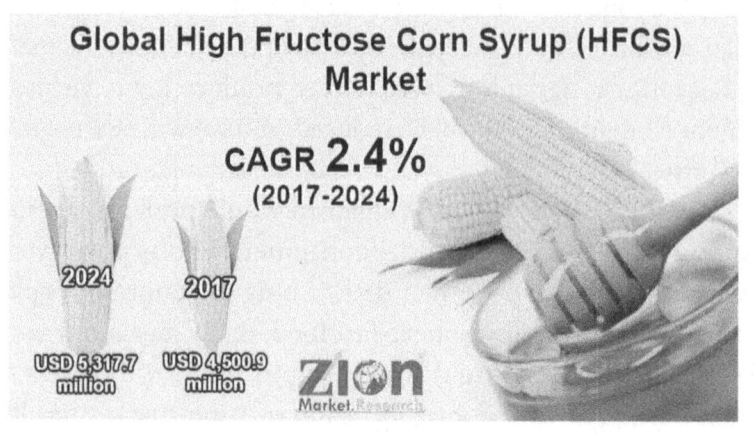

The predicted expansion of the corn syrup market

Sweetened food has become the new normal. This has contributed to a dramatic and visible increase in overweight people. However, high consumption of fructose also has other less visible and less well known side effects that create health risks. Some early evidence from a small Swiss study of children aged six to fourteen suggests that it not only leads to overweight in children, but also to smaller LDL (bad) cholesterol particle size, which is an early warning sign of risk for atherosclerosis and type 2 diabetes.[50]

High levels of fructose also affect the health of the gut. As we have seen, a healthy gut is lined with mucus. Many gut bacteria live in the mucus; some – such as lactobacillus – support the production of mucus and keep it thick, so it can act as a barrier stopping pathogenic bacteria from getting through to the endothelial cells and infecting them. Recent research also suggests the mucus also disarms pathogenic bacteria by making them less able to communicate with each other and less able to get infections off the ground.[51] However, unhealthy Western diets, including those with high levels of fructose, undermine these protective functions. They reduce the diversity of bacteria, as well as increasing pro-inflammatory bacteria in the gut. They also degrade the mucus barrier, reducing mucus thickness, allowing toxins and pathogens through.[52]

Yet governments continue to allow high fructose to saturate our food. In Europe, past restrictions have been lifted and production is predicted to rise dramatically in the next decade. In the USA, there are still massive financial subsidies for corn production for the short-term goal of making agriculture more profitable – a short-sighted strategy that mimics the addictive thinking of people reaching for a soda drink or other sweet food for comfort, discounting future effects on health and well-being. Ironically, such single-track focus on immediate profit has had disastrous economic as well as health side effects, as it has contributed to the sky-rocketing costs of healthcare for rising numbers of sufferers from diabetes and other obesity-related diseases.

Obesity and harsh parenting

There are other influences on obesity that are also rarely discussed because they are seen by some as a political hot potato: in particular, the effect of the stress of socio-economic disadvantage on parenting.

It doesn't take much imagination to appreciate that the daily grind of poverty can take a psychological toll. When life is a struggle, emotional capacity may be taken up with meeting constant challenges; there is often less time available to respond to children's unspoken emotional needs in a sensitive way. Instead, adults under pressure may use their physical power over the child to coerce the child into desired behaviours as fast as possible.

Certainly there are strong links between low socio-economic status and harsher parenting. In one national database, about 25% of low socio-economic status parents were defined as harsh parents, compared to 15% of higher socio-economic status parents – which means they swear, threaten, insult, humiliate and criticise their child.[53] Researchers have consistently found links between low income and increased use of physical punishment.[54] Some parents feel justified in using such practices. Just as with the African-American mothers who chose not to breastfeed because it 'spoils' the baby, the rationale for authoritarian parenting may be the parental belief that children must learn to deal with a harsh, unequal society from the start. As Linda Tirado put it, 'I'm not preparing our kids for a gentle world, full of interesting and stimulating experiences. I'm getting them ready to keep their damn mouths shut while some idiot tells them what to do.'[55] Low socio-economic status, teenage, or single parents have also been found to have the highest rate of 'dismissing' attachment styles designed to minimise emotional responsiveness in a harsh environment.[56]

Although there are well-documented psychological consequences of harsh parenting, an unintended and little-known consequence is that harsh or authoritarian early relationships may themselves contribute to obesity. One large study of over 37,000 children in Canada found that the child of an authoritarian parent is 44% more likely to be obese.[57] What could explain this link? One possibility is people who had over-controlling parents learn to ignore their own feelings and body signals in order to meet the parents' requirements – so they become inattentive to their own bodily cues telling them when they are hungry or when they are full.

Insecure attachment relationships in early life have also been linked to an increased risk of obesity. This type of attachment relationship can be found in any social group, but is most prevalent in low socio-economic settings, particularly where parents are young, uneducated, unsupported or depressed. Again, one very large American study found that insecurely attached two-year-olds were more likely to be obese by the time they start school aged four.[58] Speculatively, this may be in part because parents who are themselves under extreme stress are less able to help their children to manage their emotions and to regulate their states by psychological means. Poverty can bring many deep anxieties, and such states of mind are likely to make it more difficult to be responsive to a baby crying at 4 a.m. or to be attentive to a toddler's repetitive games.

Research suggests it is particularly difficult for single parents or depressed parents to manage the challenging behaviour of toddlers. Most of us can imagine the frustration of being faced with a toddler throwing food on a freshly cleaned floor or having a tantrum in a supermarket. In such situations, setting limits with firm consequences is a task that demands a high level of self-confidence and energy that the weary parent may not be able to find. Yet this is a crucial period for socialisation and developing self-regulation.[59] If this self-regulation doesn't develop well, the child may grow up into an adult less able to soothe him- or herself and, ultimately, may become more susceptible to using smoking, eating or using drugs and alcohol for this purpose.

The brain development that supports the ability to pay attention, control attention and manage heightened emotions starts very young indeed and depends greatly on the parents' own ability to pay attention to their infant. In a relaxed, secure relationship, based on consistent parental responsiveness, we are motivated to pay close attention to our mother or father's looks and gestures, and to follow the direction of the parent's gaze. This close mutual attention becomes an essential early building block for emotional self-control and self-regulation.

However, this is likely to be more difficult to achieve in disadvantaged and stressful circumstances. One startling study by Melissa Clearfield and Kelly Jedd in 2013 found that babies from low socio-economic status backgrounds consistently performed worse in various tests of attention, from as early as six months old (confirmed by repeated tests at nine and twelve months). Why would this particularly affect babies of low-income families? One possibility they mention is that nutritional deficits, such as a lack of protein, might play a part. Equally, they propose that the negative emotional atmosphere of a chronically stressed family can make babies more easily upset and less likely to want to focus on their parent's face – and so less able to let their parent guide their attention. As the authors of this study argue, it is imperative to detect these early differences in babies' capacity to pay attention, 'because it has already been established that inattention at 1 year is predictive of attentional behaviour and hyperactivity at 3.5 years'.[60]

Other evidence confirms that the strains and stresses of disadvantage can affect early brain development. Several studies have linked early poverty and low income with reduced growth of the prefrontal cortex relative to better-off babies. This starts very early, as early as one month old,[61] and five months old,[62] with differences that continue to build strongly over the crucial first three years of development and then level off. One substantial long-term prospective study in Germany by Natalie Holz and her colleagues found that poverty in the early months had a particular impact on the growth of the part of the brain involved in emotional self-regulation (the orbitofrontal pre-frontal cortex), with effects lasting into adulthood, such as difficulty with controlling impulsive behaviour.[63] Poverty later on did not have this effect.

Nurturing despite everything

Despite these potential effects of social disadvantage on the early development of attention and self-regulation, poverty is not inevitably associated with harsh parenting nor with insecure attachment.[64] A majority of parents living in conditions of economic disadvantage are still able to offer the warmth and attunement that buffers their child from stress and protects their health – perhaps because they have supportive people in their lives, or most likely because they enjoyed good regulatory relationships with their own parents.[65]

This can also affect behaviour into adolescence. People who had poor but nurturing parents –who are able to keep track of their child's activities without being excessively controlling or authoritarian – are less likely to smoke or to use drugs or other substances. Again, they are resilient people, not because of some innate quality in them but because of better emotional self-regulation and social competence.[66]

Their health is also likely to be better. Individuals who described their childhood relationship with their mother as a warm one had a normal stress response and were better regulated in adulthood,[67] while another study found that young adults who felt warmly towards their mothers showed fewer signs of systemic inflammation.[68]

While children from low socio-economic status homes are more likely to experience metabolic ill health, such as high blood pressure, insulin resistance and obesity, this is less likely when low socio-economic status mothers are warm.[69]

Clearly, both diet and psychological factors can play a role in obesity and may set up a vicious cycle. Once obesity is established, each kilo of excess fat itself generates millions of macrophages, increasing inflammation.[70] When an Australian team, led by Richard Liu, examined the evidence for a link between low socio-economic status and adult inflammation, he found a long and winding path that led from low childhood socio-economic status affecting childhood BMI, leading to high adult BMI, which in turn led to increased adult CRP.[71]

Early poverty is important for health, because it can cause stressed parenting and addictions such as smoking and poor nutrition, often leading to high BMI and obesity. In early life, these effects of poverty can then be 'embedded biologically', particularly in fetuses, babies and children under two, through passing on an obesity-prone microbiome, an altered, dysregulated, stress response and increased levels of chronic inflammation persisting into adulthood, and making serious adult physical illness more likely – even if the individual as an adult is no longer in a low socio-economic group.[72]

Is it just about the money?

In the political world, there are two stories about poverty competing for dominance. One version presents poverty as a social problem, a correctible imbalance of jobs and incomes, while the other approaches poverty as a moral failing, a form of individual dependence and failure. Each narrative leads to different solutions.

On the political right, the narrative is often moralistic and judgemental. Although, in recent times, the more tactfully named 'troubled family' concept has replaced the hostile 'lazy scrounger' trope, there are echoes of it in the view of former UK Conservative opposition leader Iain Duncan Smith, that the sources of child poverty are 'weak parenting skills, debt from financial incompetence or mental health problems'. Welfare dependency and family breakdown are seen as the result of a lack of commitment to a stable marriage,[73] and as a central factor in poverty. Certainly it is true that two out of three children growing up in poverty will have experienced family breakdown – nearly half of under fives in low-income households are not living with both parents (compared to 16% of children in higher-income households). But is this cause or effect re the stresses of poverty? And can individuals voluntarily overcome their difficulties by an act of will, as seems to be implied?

On the left, the narrative is focused on finding a remedy for unequal financial resources. These may include redistributing wealth through taxes, pursuing full-employment economic policies, action to support secure job contracts, increased minimum wage, and more social housing. As Alison Garnham of the Child Poverty Action Group put it, 'children are much more likely to be in poverty today because they have a parent who is a security guard, care worker or cleaner than a drug addict or "feckless".'[74] She rightly points to the structural factors leading to poverty that are not caused by individual choices.

However, focusing on money alone leads some champions of the economically disadvantaged to be reluctant to acknowledge that the enormous stress of poverty may indeed lead to addictions, relationship problems and difficulties in meeting the emotional needs of children. This reluctance to acknowledge the emotional fall-out of poverty can then lead, in some cases, to a resistance to the provision of psychological help for parents, which some critics have seen as intrusive, an oppressive middle-class demand for disadvantaged parents to 'parent their children out of poverty'.[75]

There is some evidence that parents with a history of difficulties may legitimately fear the power of child protection social workers to judge their parenting as inadequate and to remove their baby.[76] However, my own experience of providing such psychological help for many years to a wide range of parents and babies, many from disadvantaged backgrounds, is that when help is targeted on understanding parental difficulties and building on their strengths, parents feel better supported and more confident in their parenting. This can lead to a deeper understanding of the developmental process and more ability to respond and to give attention to their infants' emotional needs. A recent review of parenting support programmes agreed. Finnish academics, led by Kristian Wahlbeck, found strong evidence that such interventions mitigated some of the negative effects of poverty and inequality on mental health and improved children's well-being.[77]

Some of those who are wary of psychological help prefer direct cash. Indeed, there is some evidence from US studies that increasing family income by $3–4,000 dollars a year can result in some modest increases in children's cognitive development and educational attainment.[78] However, the influential economist Greg Duncan, who has spent his long academic career investigating the effects of income inequality and child poverty, believes that the impact of cash support for families in poverty varies tremendously depending on the age of the child.

Informed by the neuroscience and developmental thinking of recent years, Duncan has argued that there is a 'negligible role for income beyond age five'. In his view, cash support is most effective when targeted at pregnancy and the first years of life, when the foundations of health are laid and the capacity for self-regulation is established, which in practice underpins the ability to learn. In 2013, Duncan won a million Swiss francs to help him set up a major, long-term $17 million research study to confirm or disprove this thesis, and to find out whether or not very early cash support might have long-term benefits for the development of poor children. It is due to report over the next few years.

In the meantime, he has been an advisor to US President Biden, arguing that he should weight his 2021 expanded child tax credit in favour of the under fives. As Duncan put it, 'The fundamental difference between the children of the poor and the well-off is established by the age of five, and poorer children rarely make up the ground they've lost by then.'[79] Biden's improved tax credit was a rare success in the battle against child poverty. In Britain in the 2020s, however, child poverty continues to rise, particularly in

London and the North East. However, governments of all political persuasions still have difficulty in recognising that financial stress is not the only influence on children's health. Societies that do not support early parenting in other ways, such as providing psychological help or ensuring access to healthy food and secure housing, are also storing up problems for the future health of those children.

Conclusion

8.
Future-proofing human beings

> *'But now here were distinguished doctors and scientists arguing that the future of medicine lay in a completely different direction: get people to change their diets, control pollution, and many diseases would evaporate like snow on a sunny day. Could it be that simple?'*
>
> James Le Fanu

In recent times, 'following the science' has become a mantra used by politicians to legitimise political choices, such as during a pandemic. In practice, science is not so clear-cut. Even when there is a general consensus, there are always different interpretations of 'the science', and evidence may be contradictory or complex – particularly when there are many overlapping sources from a variety of disciplines. In addition, science may reveal unwelcome information that suggests the need for long-term planning and burdensome investment. How tempting, then, to minimise or ignore such 'inconvenient truths' – as Al Gore once memorably described the urgent need to prevent the escalating calamity of climate overheating.

Despite the provisional nature of all knowledge, decades of work in a variety of specialisms – from nutritional science, immunology, epigenetics, psychology to microbiology – has begun to firmly establish the significance of the first 1,001 days of human development in shaping future health outcomes. Scientists from a range of disciplines are helping us to understand more clearly the biological processes involved. As researchers at the University of Colorado put it, 'The complex pathways that connect diet, the microbiota, immune system development, and metabolism, particularly in early life, present exciting new frontiers for biomedical research.'[1] Such research into the biology of early development is increasingly making sense of many health issues, especially chronic illnesses that show up in later years.

Yet for some this information, too, is inconvenient, because it generates a new set of challenges and priorities. There is a real difficulty in translating these findings into effective action. We should do more than admire the exciting possibilities: we need to use research to change clinical practice and social policy. There is already much that could be done to prevent so many people from suffering the chronic illnesses of middle and old age – cardiovascular, metabolic and neuro-inflammatory – yet governments and healthcare providers as yet seem unable to commit themselves whole-heartedly to tackling them at the source, with a range of interventions in very early life. An obvious practical obstacle is the difficulty in finding extra financial resources to back preventive measures when there is so much pressure on the existing provision of healthcare. Currently, within the British NHS, prevention represents a vanishingly small proportion of its budget – around 5%.[2]

Pursuing the strategy of prevention also presents a change of emphasis for the medical profession. Potentially, it challenges current assumptions, which are, broadly speaking, based on an individualistic view of health as well as on support for the medical industrial complex. Under the sway of these ideologies, many medical professionals follow the lead of the big drug companies, private health providers and manufacturers of alcohol, nicotine and ultra-processed food, who disregard the importance of nutrition to health, and show little awareness of health as an interactive, social process particularly rooted in early life. The authority of such powerful corporate forces is difficult to question and their influence is widespread. Indeed, many 'Big Pharma' and medical technology directors and representatives have infiltrated some of the key health bodies, in the UK sitting on the boards of NICE (National Institute for Health and Care Excellence) and the MHRA (Medicines and Healthcare products Regulatory Agency). The General Medical Council itself invests considerable sums in fast food, drug companies, medical devices and private healthcare.[3] It has become commonplace for pharmaceutical corporations to make donations to NHS Trusts for 'collaborative projects', as well as making payments to individual health professionals in the form of consultancy fees or donations.[4] However, their agenda is one of selling medications, medical technologies and other health fixes for profit, goals that are unrelated to the possibility of preventing illness by addressing the wider social context.

There may also be less obvious factors involved in acknowledging the significance of early development. One may be the psychological impact of power and influence on attitudes to vulnerability. Psychotherapist Jean Knox argues that people who gain positions of power have often had to make themselves invulnerable to succeed, and may feel the need to attack in others what they fear in themselves, leading to 'the current trend in today's political culture to disparage and show contempt for any sort of frailty, disadvantage, need or dependence'.[5] This might lead to an aversion to focusing on meeting the needs of babies, the most vulnerable members of society, or to acknowledge the impact of social relationships on health. As Benjamin Perks from the UN Children's Fund put it, 'the main political discourses in our society don't do emotional. They only do economic and power.'[6]

Yet social context and health are inextricable. For example, in the USA, black women who experience the chronic stress of racial discrimination are twice as likely as white women to give birth prematurely, which puts their babies at an increased risk of future heart disease and stroke.[7] Clearly, considering heart disease and medical treatments for heart disease in isolation from social conditions does not make sense. But as Martin Marshall, then vice chair of the UK's Royal College of GPs, put it: 'The medical model is so dominant, so seductive in the health service, that unless we challenge it in a very concerted and focused way, we're not going to be able to develop an alternative.'[8]

The developmental perspective I have outlined in this book, based on an interactive view of health, is a starting point for an alternative approach to health. It recognises how human bodies and selves are shaped in every way by social communication, by the food system and by the physical environment. We are not isolated units that somehow exist 'prior to' or outside of society. We and our bodies come into being through society, through body contact, care and nourishment from other people and the environments we collectively create. Each of us grows and changes through our lifetime in response to what we encounter. This process is most intense in early life, when we are most dependent and open to others' influence, and then continues strongly throughout childhood to adolescence, which is another prime time of turbulent physical and mental change – and even on throughout adulthood, at a slower pace. Yet despite the ongoing nature of development, the most pivotal moments for lifelong health are the first 1,001 days, from conception through to the age of two, when key biological systems are being shaped through an interactive process. During this particularly concentrated developmental moment, we are most open to influences, at first mediated through our mother and her body, which passes on biochemical information about the world she is living in, and then shaped by parents and other caregivers on whom our life depends.

In a nutshell, this early period is a time when health capital is built. The most fortunate of us had healthy parents who ate a nourishing diet and who were sustained by supportive relationships with other people, from family to community – including state-funded health visitors and doctors, and effective financial safety nets. These provide the essential context in which parents are more able to be emotionally warm and responsive, able to give time and attention, as well as supporting the mother in the exclusive breastfeeding that also passes on immune protection. 'Could it be that simple?' as James Le Fanu put it.

Perhaps the goal is simple – but achieving it, less so. The challenge, in practice, is to create a supportive, pro-health environment in a profoundly unequal society, where those in positions of power are cut off from the lived experience of those who are most powerless. These – the most powerless – are the large numbers of parents who are trapped in stressful environments alongside noisy or polluted roads, or in mouldy flats, or are living with the psychological stress of daily job insecurities, or are the targets of racism, homophobia or other forms of hostility, while their physical well-being is undermined by poor diets. These are the parents who are encouraged by powerful advertising campaigns and consumer availability to favour formula milk to breastfeeding, and to eat highly processed and sweetened food. These are the parents whose conditions exhaust them and fracture their relationships, increase the risk of addictions and depression, promote obesity, and lead to bodily inflammation – all of which potentially affect the developing fetus and infant, passing on health risks instead of protections: the negative health equity that may play out over a lifetime.

Is it all down to parents? Where politics comes in

Parents, particularly mothers, may feel burdened by the weight of responsibility for their infant's health that all this implies. It is inescapable that what parents do has an enormous impact, because for the highly dependent baby, the parents *are* their environment. However, parents themselves do not exist in a vacuum but are part of the wider world. This wider environment also has an enormous impact on what parents can offer their babies. How can parents provide healthy food if it is an unaffordable luxury, while cheap mass-produced food is available on every high street? How can they give the important qualities of attention, soothing, reliability and positive warmth their babies need if they are exhausted from working long hours to keep a roof over their heads? How can they choose to live in a safe, unpolluted environment without a high income? How can they escape from the stress of poverty when business owners choose not to pay them a living wage? Politics and health are inextricably linked.

This poses a fundamental challenge. It raises questions about the current framework of our Western societies and our ability to prioritise the things that matter most. Our current economic model gives priority to making profit by any means. This has often involved overriding nature without regard for the by-products of economic activity, such as polluting rivers and seas with sewage or plastics, or triggering global warming by chopping down rainforest to produce more meat, or producing cheap food laced with sugar, which deviates from a natural diet and starts an internal war with our microbes. The system takes little responsibility for such 'externalities', which are seen as someone else's problem – or else portrayed as the choice of the consumer. Those caught up in the system often fail to acknowledge that their economic activity affects the wider social whole, ultimately including the planetary ecosystem – both of which must be sustained and kept in balance for the benefit of all. As the much loved environmentalist David Attenborough argued in his 2021 documentary *David Attenborough: A Life on Our Planet*: 'In this world, a species can only thrive when everything else around it thrives too. We can solve the problems we now face by embracing this reality. If we take care of nature, nature will take care of us. It's now time for our species to stop simply growing, and instead to establish a life on our planet in balance with nature – to start to thrive.'

The health sector does not have any greater regard for human well-being than other economic sectors: there is the same imperative to provide financial satisfaction for shareholders, even if it involves disregarding the practices that sustain health. Corporations are focused on whatever will generate most profit: supplying medical equipment, building new hospitals, developing new drugs and new surgical procedures. Businesses also find it worthwhile to invest in what the richest customers will buy, such as hair-loss medication and Viagra, rather than in those things that are most needed by the poorest areas of the world. Their role is not to ensure wider social benefits unless that contributes to profitability. Although much is made of the entrepreneurs who occasionally surprise us with wonderful new inventions, most original medical research is not the result of entrepreneurial activity but is underpinned by funding by the state, as we saw in the development of the AstraZeneca Covid-19 vaccine.[9] Indeed, big corporations in search of a profit have promoted many products over the years that have actively damaged health, blundering into the mass production of tobacco, of sugar and cheap high-fructose corn syrup, of diesel petrol and formula milk, drenching the food we eat with pesticides to increase production volumes, allowing patients to become addicted to the painkiller Oxycontin – to name just a few colossal errors that have only been corrected with the greatest reluctance, after much obstruction and denial.

Under the current power structures in democratic societies, politicians act as if they are relatively powerless to regulate such corporate activities. In part this is because of their ideological convictions about the 'free' market, but also, more mundanely, because they often rely on the goodwill of rich donors, usually from the corporate world, to fund their political activities and their election campaigns. Although politicians know that air pollution causes heart and lung disease, and contributes to obesity, governments remain unwilling to challenge corporations who want to continue to build new roads, new airports and who resist meeting legal targets for air quality. In a global market, they live in fear that such corporations will take jobs elsewhere, leaving an impoverished home economy.

Instead of making stringent demands on corporations to protect our health, politicians propose in hope rather than expectation that corporations should be trusted to act with social responsibility. Yet as food campaigner Michele Simon points out, quoting Joel Bakan's book *The Corporation*, 'No one would seriously suggest that individuals should regulate themselves, that laws against murder, assault and theft are unnecessary because people are socially responsible. Yet oddly, we are asked to believe that corporate persons – institutional psychopaths who lack any sense of moral conviction and who have the power and motivation to cause harm and devastation in the world – should be left free to govern themselves.'[10]

Another limiting factor is the inevitable temptation, in a political system focused on acquiring or keeping power in the short-term, to restrict legislation to short-term measures that the public will accept. These rarely produce effective prevention, which demands long-term planning and investment – especially unpopular investment that requires higher taxes. Prevention of future ill health or of climate overheating brings no instant gratification, even though both are urgently necessary. This is unlikely to change until the public – that is to say, all of us – develops more faith in long-term thinking and gives up the desire for quick fixes.[11]

Currently, many people have little faith in collective solutions. Instead, they pursue personal control and individual solutions. In particular, the individualism promoted by capitalism leads people to become emotionally attached to the mirage that economic growth will 'trickle down', bringing them greater prosperity and the opportunity to improve their own lives and those of their children – perhaps by living in better areas, or by avoiding dependence on inadequate public provision and being able to pay for privileged access to healthcare. Such aspirations are perhaps why so many admire the super-rich despite their excesses.

Health providers also focus on urging people to take individual responsibility for their health rather than addressing the wider and more intractable social determinants of health. It is currently fashionable to talk about messaging 'hard to reach' people through social media, to engage them in a 'dialogue' about their health: to encourage individuals to smoke less, eat a Mediterranean diet and exercise more. While such increased awareness and support to develop healthier habits can only be helpful, this approach on its own fails to recognise or address the deep-rooted psychological reasons why people develop unhealthy habits and addictions, as well as failing to recognise the early origins of many health problems, or the effect of widening inequalities in society.

The individualistic ideology encourages us to believe that anyone can have a long and healthy life if they work hard, do not overeat, work out in the gym and so on – that our 'lifestyle' is our choice, and we can choose to be healthy. However, our health prospects are not as much under our control as many believe. As we have seen, health inequality starts at conception. While lifestyle behaviours clearly can play a part in the unfolding of chronic illnesses, they often act as the 'second hit' that triggers the risks already set up by a shaky foundation. As Neal Halfon, professor of paediatrics at UCLA, summed it up: 'Many health conditions are disorders of development.'[12] Mothers (and, to a lesser extent, fathers) pass on their own state of health and their own stress levels during pregnancy – and postnatal parenting completes our basic physiological and emotional tool-kit. A developmental perspective shows how later opportunities are constrained by earlier events; while technically 'free', the individual cannot choose to have a robust immune system if this has not been established during early development, just as individuals who aspire to a life like Bill Gates' do not all get his head start by inheriting a million-dollar trust fund.

Whatever difference individual correctives – if undertaken early enough, or consistently enough – may make, individual efforts are not enough to have a large impact on the health of a whole society. Individuals can't address the structural underpinnings of poor health, such as the stresses of low income, of homelessness, pollution or violence, nor can they ensure that all parents get support to enable them to provide the thoughtful and protective parenting that underpins good mental and physical health. Above all, individual efforts cannot bring about the sustaining social networks that really matter most.

Too many old people?

Even politicians who want to prioritise the collective health of their own population are increasingly caught in a trap because the demographics are shifting. Changes in the way we work and live have dramatically affected life expectancy, increasing demands for healthcare. Looking backwards to the conditions of life in the nineteenth and earlier twentieth centuries, most people back then were involved in physically demanding manual labour, and often struggled to get enough food; their bodies were soon worn out and their lives tended to be short. By the latter part of the twentieth century, a new economic era was unfolding, in which sedentary occupations had become the norm in developed countries and mass-produced high calorie food was available to all. People began to live longer. Combined with a falling birth rate, this led to a dramatic increase in the number of old people relative to younger people, and current projections are that these numbers will escalate further. The fear is that this will lead to an unmanageable bill for healthcare.

Certainly, chronic ill health is very costly. According to one recent UK government document, the total cost of illness-related absence from work and lost productivity costs our economy at least £100 billion a year,[13] while a similar report in the USA suggested it loses employers $576 billion a year.[14] Much absence from work is due to coughs, colds, back pain and depression as well as chronic illnesses. However, the biggest health treatment costs are increasingly generated by the chronic diseases of older age. These soak up a large proportion of NHS funding in the UK. According to the Department of Health's 2011 website, the approximate figure is around 70% of 'the primary and acute care budget'.[15]

This growing epidemic of chronic ill health is not inevitable. Understanding the underlying processes that lead to the familiar litany of illnesses – type 2 diabetes, obesity, cardiovascular disease, neuroinflammatory conditions and cancer – could lead to a new focus on good early nurturing to reduce these health risks. Much more funding could be directed to supporting pregnant women and families with babies and toddlers, reducing stress and improving nutrition at the start of life – as well as seriously tackling the unhealthy food system based on processed food. Providing better support for breastfeeding should be a central plank in a preventive approach. UNICEF calculates that increasing breastfeeding in the UK would not only reduce infant hospital admissions, saving millions of pounds, but would also result in fewer breast cancer cases and further millions of expenditure on care for women so afflicted.[16] With a new, preventive focus, these health vulnerabilities would diminish, and older age outcomes could be improved. More older people could remain in good health, potentially continuing to contribute to the economy as well as making fewer demands on public health services.

Medical model

Unfortunately, the medical profession does not seem to have taken on board the significance of early development. It remains relatively entrenched in a much narrower medical model focused on the mechanics of the body and how it malfunctions due to genetic vulnerability or when some physical or chemical event, such as an infection or injury, disturbs the norm. The current medical model has not fully adapted to the rise of slowly evolving chronic conditions rooted in early developmental processes, nor embraced an understanding of the body in its ecology, affected by nutrition and social relationships.

Currently, few doctors and nurses are trained in the relevance of early nutrition for health, or in the role played by the microbiome. It is simply not an important part of the curriculum. As Saman Vareki, a Canadian oncologist working on the role of diet in cancer, put it, 'significant numbers of both clinicians and scientists discount the role of the microbiome in health and disease'.[17]

Likewise, medical trainees are rarely encouraged to recognise the importance of psychological and social impacts, particularly those related to early development and early trauma, let alone take into account the impact on health of the broader social stresses of marginalisation, poverty and racism. As campaigning GP Malcolm Kendrick put it in his inimitable style, 'I recognise that it is difficult for the medical profession to do a great deal about social health, it is not their area, they are taught little about it. It is far easier to stick to clever things like managing type IV tubular acidosis in chronic renal failure. More difficult to look at the "soft factors".'[18] As a result, many medics find themselves unwittingly co-opted into the priorities dictated by big corporations, with their pursuit of marvellously sophisticated surgical procedures to remove tumours and repair failing body parts, genomic advances and new drug treatments to suppress symptoms.

And, indeed, business is booming for 'Big Pharma'. Prescription volumes in the UK have been rising annually; in 2017–2018, 26% of the adult population received at least one prescription a year. By 2021–2022, the cost of these prescription medicines had reached £17.2 billion.[19] In the USA, prescription volumes are even higher; sales of drugs to treat cancer alone have increased by 60% since 2013. This is partly thanks to the 1983 Orphan Drug Act in the USA, which offered financial incentives to develop drugs for rare conditions with only a small market (such as rare cancers), bringing more drug treatments onto the market, often at an astronomical price. Other pharmaceutical innovations are also exploring ever more personalised drug treatments. The exciting 'cutting edge' is seen as genomic testing, which offers the prospect of tailoring drug treatments to suit a particular individual's genes, or to predict which patients might have adverse reactions to particular drugs, such as chemotherapy.[20]

These advances are wonderful for the individuals who benefit. However, they have taken a dominant place in thinking about health, leaving little space for consideration of the social determinants of health and illness.

Prevention

Prevention is increasingly defined in hi-tech terms – for example, being able to sequence an individual's genome in order to predict an individual's risk of developing particular diseases such as cancers, enabling earlier detection and 'new treatment options'.[21] As outlined in a recent policy document, the UK government argues that it is genomics that will enable us to understand 'what causes illness and infectious disease', as if health outcomes depend on an individual's DNA alone. But as we have seen, the search for common genetic variants linked to non-communicable diseases (NCDs) – those conditions that you cannot catch from other people – has come up empty.[22] Few diseases are caused by single genes; most complex diseases involve many different genes interacting with their environment. Even those who do possess 'risky' genes that make them more susceptible to particular forms of illness do not automatically become ill, since their DNA does not control their cells; as Gilbert Gottlieb put it, 'genes can't turn themselves on and off'.[23]

Although each person has a unique collection of genes, whether or not they are expressed is primarily driven by the individual's environment – including their diet, stress levels and exposure to pollutants. What matters most is the kind of social world they find themselves in. Most of us have genes that offer the makings of a happy and healthy life.

A different approach to prevention throws the spotlight back on the social world and the environment we collectively create. While medical advances through surgical techniques and new drugs are undeniably impressive responses to a malfunctioning body, the evidence of the past tells us that the factors that have had the greatest impact on *preventing* ill health have been less glamorous, practical measures, such as mass vaccination programmes as well as infrastructure achievements, such as clean water supply and the building of sewers. These have been highly successful in reducing or even eliminating many of the infectious diseases that were the greatest threat to human health in the past.

However, in the modern post-war period, new health threats have taken centre stage. Apart from the challenge of new viral pandemics, the dominant health issues of our own era are now the NCDs, such as metabolic diseases like type 2 diabetes, as well as neuro-inflammatory conditions, chronic obstructive pulmonary disease (COPD), some cancers and cardiovascular disease. These pose new challenges for prevention.

As demands on health services grow, one group of public health academics has even begun to argue that the goal of health policy should not be to pursue the unattainable goal of health for all. Instead, the goal should be to promote the individual's 'ability to adapt and self-manage . . . in the face of social, physical and emotional challenges'.[24] Instead of giving fresh impetus to prevention via tackling the social scourges of child neglect and abuse, stressful inequality, an unhealthy food system, pollution and climate overheating, the implication is that these conditions are accepted as facts of life to which the individual must adapt.

Indeed, the healthy resilience and adaptability this group of academics advocates largely depends on positive social experiences, particularly in early life. Those very soothing systems we rely on to meet threats and challenges in a healthy way are built from social experiences of good early care and nutrition.

In a situation where there is a critical lack of funding for health care, it is tempting to hand responsibility back to the individual, rather than to tackle overwhelmingly difficult questions about priorities and how we deal with social problems. Our current mindset favours tolerance of an unhealthy, careless and unsustainable way of life and then, when chickens come home to roost, looks to technology to fix the problems that arise (with medications for stress and nutrition-related disease, or geo-engineering for climate overheating). Instead, we could focus on how to prevent such predicaments from arising by intervening in the earliest phases of development rather than waiting for symptoms to appear. However, this would redefine health as a social issue, one demanding foresight and state investment in better nutrition, better care and in reducing stress, particularly for young families.

A greater investment in more effective prevention of ill health does not mean that our current 'illness service' should be downgraded. Of course we want our health problems, our chronic and life-threatening illnesses, to be fixed. The painful knee, the cancerous tumour, the respiratory distress are all urgent; nothing is more important when you are suffering. I desperately want there to be a pill that will cure Parkinson's. We still need an effective illness service to treat our symptoms. However, we also need to reduce our dependency on expensive drug medications and to take more effective action to protect the next generations from needless ill health.

How can we ensure better health for the next generation?

The work summarised in this book suggests we should put much more emphasis on prevention by investing heavily in the first 1,001 days of development. It suggests that we should sharpen our focus on pregnancy and postnatal care to ensure all new humans have the health capital they need to prevent them from developing the chronic illnesses that could blight their later years and burden health care systems. Currently we are going in the opposite direction, actually reducing spending on maternal care during pregnancy and post-natal care.

There is a crisis in maternity services, which, in the UK, receive a declining and tiny percentage of the NHS budget (currently somewhere in the region of 2%). The chronic shortage of midwives has been described by Birte Harlev Lam, executive director of the Royal College of Midwives, as 'a black hole at the centre of our maternity services where more money and staff should be'.[25] Likewise, the Public Health Grant paid to Local Authorities that funds health visitors has been cut substantially and there is a shortage of health visitors, equating to a loss of 40% of practitioners since 2015.[26]

Paradoxically, the arguments for investing in pregnancy and postnatal care have become well established and well made over the last two decades. In the UK, both charitable and state-funded projects to support parents and babies have multiplied – OXPIP, Sure Start, the Healthy Child Programme, Start for Life, A Better Start, Best Beginnings and so on. Yet, despite these efforts, funding remains inadequate and insecure. Indeed, public spending on early years services, including Sure Start, has decreased by 39% since 2015.[27]

There are a number of practical steps that could be taken. Looking at the bigger picture, measures to address socio-economic deprivation, particularly in families with young children, are an important plank in reducing stress. Longterm, decent housing and jobs are essential to creating a secure basis for family life. Temporary financial support is also crucial for families with babies and toddlers. In particular, long-lasting, well-paid maternity and paternity leave can make a huge contribution to reducing parental stress and improving nutrition for babies. It can make it easier to breastfeed babies by relieving the pressure on mothers to return to work. As things stand in the UK, state-funded maternity pay is currently only £184 a week, pro rata equivalent to an annual salary of around £9,569 (or less if the mother normally earns less than this), and is only available for about eight months (after the first six weeks at a higher rate). These meagre sums don't offer a viable alternative to a working income.

Contrast this provision with that provided by most Scandinavian countries, where parental leave is closer to 80% of pay throughout (which, on the current average UK woman's annual income of £29,842, would be £23,873). In Sweden, this level of support is available for around sixteen months and can be shared between both parents, with the side benefit of promoting parental gender equality and fathers' involvement with their babies. Fathers can also take up to thirty paid days off in the first year after the birth, any time their partner needs support. Such social measures have a real impact on parental health, for example by reducing mothers' prescriptions for anxiety medication by 26%.[28] Generous maternity and paternity leave also helps to support relationships between parents and babies. A recent study found that the longer the maternity leave taken, the better the quality of interactions between mother and baby, and the more likely they are to enjoy a secure attachment relationship.[29]

However, financial interventions are unlikely to be effective on their own. Recent research found that the lasting effect of adverse childhood experiences (ACEs) on health are independent

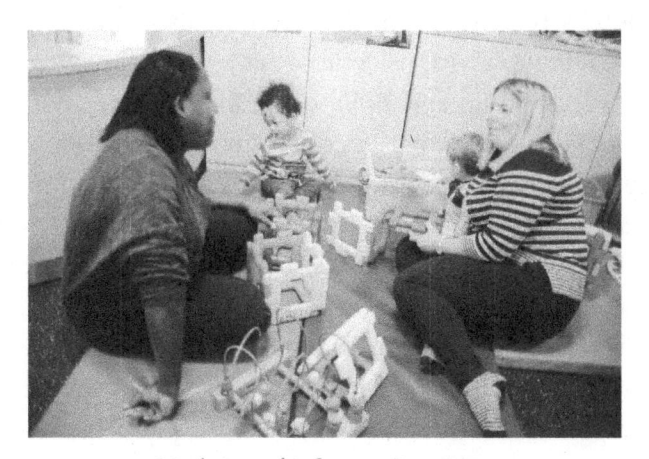

Mothers and infants at Sure Start

of socio-economic factors.[30] Although many factors play a part, some evidence suggests that the quality of early relationships is a major factor.

While financial stress can certainly be a factor in triggering harsh or neglectful parenting, parenting practices are also influenced by negative and often unconscious patterns of behaviour formed by parents' own childhood experiences. These 'ghosts in the nursery' were a regular feature of my clinical work with parents and babies over many years. For example, I worked with a young mother called Eddie, whose own mother had labelled her a difficult baby and left her feeling bad as a child. Eddie had not dealt with these feelings from childhood and brought her long-suppressed anger with her mother into her relationship with her new baby, Noah. She attempted to force him to do what she wanted, as her mother had done with her (the 'training' model of parenting again). In response, Noah's muscles were chronically tensed and he regularly sicked up, making him hard to cuddle or enjoy. In fact, Eddie guiltily confessed that she 'hated' him.

Another common theme in my clinical practice was an underlying fear of not being good enough and being rejected by the baby. Bella, another mother I worked with, had past experiences that led her to fear this. Her baby read her anxious body language and responded by recoiling from her, avoiding eye contact and rarely smiling, leading to a vicious cycle of mutual dislike.

Parents like Eddie and Bella often feel intense shame about their feelings and can experience great relief and hope when they are helped through psychotherapy to develop a compassionate understanding of some of the roots of their difficulties with their babies. I have witnessed many transformed relationships as a result of supportive parent–infant psychotherapies, such as Watch, Wait and Wonder, or Video Interaction Guidance (VIG), that draw attention to moments of sensitivity and connection between parent and baby. These can give parents greater confidence, warmth and understanding of their baby's needs.

Nurturing the nurturers is a key strategy to protect infant health and well-being.

Many of these goals could be delivered by setting up young family community health centres in every neighbourhood, much like the UK's Sure Start centres of the early 2000s, so cruelly decimated by a policy of economic austerity. Unlike Sure Start, which had a wider remit, these might be most effective for future health if targeted primarily at families in the first 1,001 days. Currently, a new scheme in the UK called Start For Life, offering funding to Local Authorities to provide support for breastfeeding and early parenting at 'Family Hubs', is being piloted. However, its future is uncertain. In theory, such local neighbourhood centres could make a real difference, particularly if they are psychologically 'owned' by local people. They could potentially help ensure all pregnant women have access to nutritious food by providing a supply of fresh vegetables, a café, even cooking lessons for those who want them. Meeting other new families would support community friendship networks, which can help to reduce stress. Practical advice and help – for example, to manage debt and housing problems – could also be offered alongside the targeted specialist psychological support I have described. Importantly, services based at these centres should be free and universally available to all those who need them. More traumatised families, particularly parents in destructive or violent relationships, very young parents or those whose lives are chaotic and who are unlikely to seek out professional help, may need more intensive help. There is an effective, well-researched programme from the USA called the Family Nurse Partnership that could be made more widely available. This programme establishes a supportive relationship between a psychologically trained nurse, midwife or health visitor and an 'at risk' family, reaching out to 'hard to reach' parents through home visits from pregnancy until the baby is two years old. In the UK, the programme was first piloted in 2007, but in this country has been limited to teenage mothers. Like so many early intervention services, it is not universally available as yet but depends on particular local commissioners choosing to offer the service.

Much greater investment in the first 1,001 days would start to turn the tide to protect our health services from being overwhelmed by future NCDs. Its underlying purpose would be to aim to ensure the next generations are not exposed to the early stresses that can lead to hypersensitive stress responses and the bacterial imbalances and chronic inflammation that create future health problems. At the same time, a wider recognition that early relationships have biological consequences offers the best chance of developing strategies to minimise those consequences as far as possible, and to provide a more compassionate response to the many who are affected.

For me and my generation, these 'future' health problems have already started to arrive. Aside from the cool statistics, I now begin to appreciate what these illnesses actually feel like and the many varieties of distress as mental and physical health disintegrates. NCD symptoms can include chronic pain, chest pain, heart palpitations, fainting, falling, tiredness, and difficulty with the basic functions of the body: difficulty walking, frequent urinating, constipation, trouble swallowing and speaking, dimming vision, impaired memory and thinking, even breathing. The slow erosion of faculties in normal ageing is overtaken by an accelerated form of ageing on speed-dial.

I remember the last time I saw my friend Dave. We met for lunch in a pub in Essex with our dogs. Dave was on good form, cracking jokes and bringing his usual empathy to bear as we updated each other on our lives. After lunch we set off for a short walk with the dogs.

However, although willing himself to overcome his COPD (chronic obstructive pulmonary disease) symptoms, Dave soon became breathless, struggling even to walk across the car park to his car and his portable oxygen. His failing body was no longer in sync with his spirited self and his life was prematurely cut short a few months later.

The more I have come to understand about the early factors that might have influenced my own health in later life, the sadder I feel that this information was not available sooner. My parents did not know – nor was it public knowledge – and my own awareness has been equally belated. Although I have paid reasonable attention to my own diet and exercise over many years, I now realise that such efforts were no match for the deep roots of potential ill health set up in my first 1,001 days. Greater awareness, however, might have led me to make different choices. I hope the information in this book will enable others to understand their own history so that they can seek screening, treatment or other preventive measures to counter stress and inflammation in order to protect their health.

We could reduce the misery for future generations. Much has changed in recent decades, which suggests it is time to re-evaluate. The growing understanding of epigenetics, of nutrition, the microbiome and of the role of stress and inflammation on health takes us in a new direction, pointing to the case for a developmental perspective on health. This knowledge increasingly directs us back to our beginnings, to the importance of our mammalian selves and those drives to hold and cherish and nurture our babies with good food and good care in the widest sense. This is how we will grow healthy people who have robust regulatory systems that can withstand the inevitable stresses of life and defeat the pathogens around us.

Care is central to health. It is not an optional extra, a luxury for the lucky few. Warm, attentive relationships that support good physiological regulation make it possible for health to flourish. Equally, care for the wider environment and good regulation of the public sphere is also necessary for children's health and well-being, allowing them to thrive. Effective social regulation that prevents unsafe housing, polluted air, contaminated rivers, an overheating climate and food adulterated by sugar is crucial, yet still so difficult for societies in thrall to ideals of individual freedom to make money. As W. M. Thackeray put it in his novel *Vanity Fair*, written in an earlier phase of capitalism, this remains 'a world where everyone is striving for what is not worth having'.[31]

Health, on the other hand, is worth having.

Notes

Introduction

1 Gerhardt, S., *Why Love Matters: How Affection Shapes a Baby's Brain* (Routledge, 2004, 2014).
2 Bandura, A., 'Social cognitive theory: an agentic perspective', *Annual Review of Psychology*, 52 (2001), pp. 1–26.
3 Dubos, R., *Man Adapting* (Yale University Press, 1965, 1980).
4 Zouikr, I., and Karshikoff, B., 'Lifetime modulation of pain system via neuroimmune and neuroendocrine interactions', *Frontiers in Immunology*, 8 (2017), p. 276.
5 Rowitch, D., 'This idea must die: Paediatrics is about jabs, broken arms and nosebleeds', *CAM* 90 (2020).

PART ONE

Health Stories

1. Germs and genes

1 Tan, S. and Rogers, L. 'Louis Pasteur (1822–1895): the germ theorist', *Singapore Medical Journal*, 48 (1): 4 (2007).
2 Frieden, T., 'Exclusive: Center for Disease Control Chief Frieden: How to end America's growing opioid epidemic', Fox News (17 December 2016).
3 Mikulic, M., 'Global spending on medicines 2010–2027', Statista (22 May 2024); Gusovsky, D., 'Americans consume vast majority of the world's opioids', CNBC (27 Apr 2016).

Notes

4 Weindling, P., 'Julian Huxley and the continuity of eugenics in twentieth-century Britain', *Journal of Modern European History*, 10:4 (2012), pp. 480–499.

5 Bouche, T., and Rivard, L., 'America's Hidden History: the Eugenics Movement', Scitable, Nature Education (2014); Krisch, J., 'When Racism Was a Science', *New York Times* (13 October 2014).

6 'Genetics [as a risk factor for breast cancer]', Breastcancer.org/risk/risk-factors/genetics (updated 9 March 2024).

7 Wade, N., 'A decade later, genetic map yields few new cures', *New York Times* (12 June 2010).

8 Rose, S., 'School achievement isn't just in your genes', *New Scientist* (18 October 2013).

9 Bruu Carver, R. et al, 'Young adults' belief in genetic determinism', *PLoS One*, 12:1 (23 Jan 2017); Kampourakis, K. et al, 'Genetics and society: educating scientifically literate citizens', *Science and Education*, 23 (2014) pp. 251–8.

10 Haggbloom, S. et al, 'The most eminent 100 psychologists of the 20th century', *Review of General Psychology*, 6:2 (2002), pp. 139–52.

11 Plomin, R., *Blueprint: How DNA Makes Us Who We Are* (Allen Lane, 2018).

12 www.youtube.com/watch?v=FptGxaxJyms

13 Plomin, R., *Blueprint*.

14 Buss, A., and Plomin, R., *Temperament: Early Developing Personality Traits* (Taylor & Francis, 1984).

15 Hernandez, L., and Blazer, D. (eds), *Genes, Behaviour and the Social Environment* (The National Academies Press, 2006).

16 Guttinger, S., and Dupre, J., 'Genomics and Postgenomics', *Stanford Encyclopedia of Philosophy* (2016).

17 Moore, D.S., *The Developing Genome* (Oxford University Press, 2015).

18 Van de Vijver, G. et al, 'Epigenetics: a challenge for genetics, evolution and development?', *Annals of the New York Academy of Sciences*, 981 (Dec 2002), pp. 1–6.

19 Chalfun, G. et al, 'Perinatal stress and methylation of the NR3C1 gene in newborns: systematic review', *Epigenetics*, 17:9 (2002), pp. 1003–19.

20 Lester, B. et al, 'Epigenetic programming by maternal behaviour in the human infant', *Pediatrics*, 142:4 (Oct 2018); Pickles, A. et al, 'Prenatal anxiety, maternal stroking in infancy, and symptoms of emotional and behavioural disorders at 3.5 years', *European Child and Adolescent Psychiatry*, 26:3 (Mar 2017), pp. 325–34.

21 Weaver, I. et al, 'Reversal of maternal programming of stress responses in adult offspring through methyl supplementation: altering epigenetic marking later in life', *Journal of Neuroscience*, 25:47 (23 Nov 2005), pp. 11045–54.

22 Aggarwal, R. et al, 'Natural compounds: role in reversal of epigenetic changes', *Biochemistry* (Moscow), 80:8 (Aug 2015), pp. 972–89; Campbell, C., 'Cancer prevention and treatment by wholistic nutrition', *Journal of Natural Sciences*, 3:10 (Oct 2017).

23 Fiorito, G. et al, 'Social adversity and epigenetic aging: a multi-cohort study on socioeconomic differences in peripheral blood DNA methylation', *Scientific Reports*, 7:16266 (24 Nov 2017); McGuinness, D., 'Socioeconomic status is associated with epigenetic differences in the pSoBid cohort', *International Journal of Epidemiology*, 41:1 (Feb 20120, pp. 151–60.

24 Ruehlmann, A. et al, 'Epigenome-wide meta-analysis of prenatal maternal stressful events and newborn DNA methylation', *Molecular Psychiatry*, 28 (Mar 2023), pp. 5090–5100.

25 Moore, D.S., *The Developing Genome*.

26 Ibid.

27 Freeman, G., 'Biodesign for the Bioeconomy', Synthetic Biology Strategic Plan 2016 Launch, 24 February 2016 (accessed at vimeo.com/157133305).

28 Ibid.

29 LaMotte, S., 'Alzheimer's: the disease that could bankrupt medicare', CNN (7 March 2017).

2. Growing a person: a social, interactive view of health

1 Robinson, M., 'President Obama and Marilynne Robinson: a Conversation—II', *New York Review of Books* (19 November 2015).
2 Cooley, C., *Human Nature and the Social Order* (Charles Scribners and Sons, 1902).
3 Drummond, J. and Wilbraham, A., *The Englishman's Food: A History of Five Centuries of English Diet* (Jonathan Cape, 1939).
4 Adams, C., 'History of Health Visiting', *Nursing in Practice*, 68 (Sept/Oct 2012).
5 White House Conference for Child Health and Protection 1930 (Smuts, 2006).
6 Stewart, J., 'The scientific claims of British child guidance, 1918–45', *British Journal for the History of Science*, 42:3 (Sep 2009), pp. 407–32.
7 Bowlby, J., 'Forty-four juvenile thieves: their characters and home-life', *The International Journal of Psychoanalysis*, 25 (1944), pp. 19–53.
8 Karen, R., *Becoming Attached* (Oxford University Press, 1998).
9 Bronfenbrenner, U. and Morris, P., 'The ecology of developmental processes' in Damon, W. and Lerner, R.M. (eds.), *Handbook of Child Psychology: Theoretical Models of Human Development* (John Wiley & Sons, 1998).
10 Silva, P., 'The Dunedin Multidisciplinary Child Development Study: an introductory overview, some findings and preliminary recommendations', University of Otago Archive, (1978).
11 Jerome Kagan (1984), quoted in Sroufe, A. et al, 'Conceptualizing the Role of Early Experience: Lessons from the Minnesota Longitudinal Study', *Developmental Review*, 30:1 (Mar 2010), pp. 36–51.
12 Sroufe, A., 'Conceptualizing the Role of Early Experience'.
13 Boyce, T. and Kobor, M., 'Development and the epigenome: the "synapse" of gene- environment interplay', *Developmental Science*, 18:1 (Jan 2015), pp. 1–23.
14 Sroufe, A., 'The concept of development in developmental psychopathology', *Child Development Perspectives*, 3:3 (Dec 2009), pp. 178–83.

15 Hartley, C. and Lee, F., 'Sensitive periods in affective development: nonlinear maturation of fear learning', *Neuropsychopharmacology*, 40:1 (Jul 2014), pp. 50–60.
16 Bush, N. et al, 'Mechanisms underlying the association between early life adversity and physical health', *Psychosomatic Medicine*, 78:9 (Nov/Dec 2016), pp. 1114–19.
17 Hartley, C. and Lee, F., 'Sensitive periods in affective development'.
18 Bruer, J., *The Myth of the First Three Years* (Simon & Schuster, 1999).
19 Weisleder, A. and Fernald, A., 'Talking to children matters: early language experience strengthens processing and builds vocabulary', *Psychological Science*, 24:11 (Nov 2013), pp. 2143–52.
20 Meins, E. and Fernyhough, C., 'Linguistic acquisitional style and mentalising development: the role of maternal mind-mindedness', *Cognitive Development*, 14:3 (Jul–Sep 1999), pp. 363–80.
21 Kotas, M. and Medzhitov, R., 'Homeostasis, inflammation and disease susceptibility', *Cell*, 160:5 (2016), pp. 816–27; Torday, J., 'Homeostasis as the mechanism of evolution', *Biology*, 4:3 (Sep 2015), pp. 573–90.
22 Schore, A., 'Early interpersonal neurobiological assessment of attachment and autistic spectrum disorders', *Frontiers in Psychology*, 5 (2014), article 1049; Troller-Renfree, S. and Fox, N., 'Sensitive periods of development: Implications for risk and resilience' in Luby, J. (ed.), *Handbook of Preschool Mental Health* (Guilford Publications, 2017).
23 Hartley, C. and Lee, F., 'Sensitive periods in affective development'.
24 'Tuning in: parents of young children tell us what they think, know and need', Zero to Three, National Parent Survey Report (2015).
25 Maguire-Jack, K. et al, 'Spanking and child development during the first five years of life', *Child Development*, 83:6 (Nov 2012), pp. 1960–77.
26 Heilmann, A. et al, 'Physical punishment and child outcomes: a narrative review of prospective studies', *The Lancet*, 398:10297 (Jul 2021), pp. 355–64.
27 Doom, J. and Gunnar, M., 'Stress physiology and developmental psychopathology: past, present and future', *Developmental Psychopathology*, 25:4:2 (Nov 2013), pp. 1359–73.

28 Tyrka, A. et al, 'Childhood adversity and epigenetic regulation of glucocorticoid signalling genes', *Developmental Psychopathology*, 28:4:2 (Nov 2016), pp. 1319–31.

29 Liu, P. and Nusslock, R., 'How stress gets under the skin: early life adversity and glucocorticoid receptor epigenetic regulation', *Current Genomics*, 19:8 (Dec 2018), pp. 653–64, 2018; Tyrka, A. et al, 'Childhood adversity and epigenetic regulation of glucocorticoid signalling genes'; Doom, J. and Gunnar, M., 'Stress physiology and developmental psychopathology'; Mulligan, C. and Friedman, J., 'Maternal modifiers of the infant gut microbiota – metabolic consequences', *Journal of Endocrinology*, 235:1 (Oct 2017), pp. R1–R12; McGowan, P. and Matthews, S., 'Prenatal stress, glucocorticoids, and developmental programming of the stress response', *Endocrinology*, 159:1 (Jan 2018), pp. 69–82; Houtepen, L. et al, 'Genome-wide DNA methylation levels and altered cortisol stress reactivity following childhood trauma in humans', *Nature Communications*, 7 (2016), article 10967.

30 Archer, T. et al, 'Neurogenetics and epigenetics in impulsive behaviour: impact on reward circuitry', *Journal of Genetic Syndromes and Gene Therapy*, 3:3 (May 2012), p. 115.

31 Doom, J. and Gunnar, M., 'Stress physiology and developmental psychopathology'; Maniam, J. et al, 'Early-life stress, HPA axis adaptation, and mechanisms contributing to later health outcomes', *Frontiers in Endocrinology*, 5:73 (May 2014); McLaughlin, K. et al, 'Causal effects of the early caregiving environment on development of stress response systems in children', *Proceedings of the National Academy of Sciences of the USA*, (PNAS), 112:18 (May 2015), pp. 5637–42; Parent, J. et al, 'Dynamic stress-related epigenetic regulation of the glucocorticoid receptor gene promoter during early development: the role of child maltreatment', *Development and Psychopathology*, 29:5 (Dec 2017), pp. 1635–48.

32 Lovallo, W. et al, 'Lifetime adversity leads to blunted stress axis reactivity: studies from the Oklahoma Family Health Patterns Project', *Biological Psychiatry*, 71:4 (Feb 2012), pp. 344–9; Voellmin, A. et al,

'Blunted endocrine and cardiovascular reactivity in young healthy women reporting a history of childhood adversity', *Psychoneuroendocrinology*, 51 (Jan 2015), pp. 58–67.

33 Essex, M. et al, 'Epigenetic vestiges of early developmental adversity: childhood stress exposure and DNA methylation in adolescence', *Child Development*, 84:1 (Jan/Feb 2013), pp. 58–75.

34 Kanherkar, R. et al, 'Epigenetics across the human lifespan', *Frontiers in Cell and Developmental Biology*, 2 (2014), p. 49.

35 Zucchi, F. et al, 'The secret language of destiny: stress imprinting and transgenerational origins of disease', *Frontiers in Genetics*, 3 (2012); Archer, T. et al, 'Neurogenetics and epigenetics in impulsive behaviour: impact on reward circuitry'.

36 Bazopoulou, D. et al, 'Developmental ROS individualizes organismal stress resistance and lifespan', *Nature*, 576 (Dec 2019), pp. 301–5.

37 Lester, B. et al, 'Epigenetic programming by maternal behaviour in the human infant'.

38 Shonkoff, J. et al, 'The lifelong effects of early childhood adversity and toxic stress', *American Academy of Pediatrics*, 129:1 (Jan 2012), e232–46.

39 Schulkin, J., 'Social allostasis: anticipatory regulation of the internal milieu', *Frontiers in Evolutionary Neuroscience*, 2 (Jan 2011), p. 111.

40 Porges, S. and Furman, E., 'The early development of the autonomic nervous system provides a neural platform for social behaviour: a polyvagal perspective', *Infant and Child Development*, 20:1 (2011), pp. 106–118.

41 Van den Bergh, B. et al, 'Antenatal maternal anxiety is related to HPA-axis dysregulation and self-reported depressive symptoms in adolescence: a prospective study of the fetal origins of depressed mood', *Neuropsychopharmacology*, 33:3 (Feb 2008), pp. 536–45; Juruena, M. et al, 'The role of early life stress in HPA axis and anxiety', *Anxiety Disorders* (2020), pp. 141–53.

42 Miller, G. et al, 'Psychological stress in childhood and susceptibility to the chronic diseases of aging: moving towards a model of behavioural

and biological mechanisms', *Psychological Bulletin*, 137:6 (Nov 2011), pp. 959–97.

43 Hong, H. et al, 'Chronic stress effects on tumor: pathway and mechanism', *Frontiers in Oncology*, 11 (Dec 2021), article 738252.

44 Ménard, C. et al, 'Immune and neuroendocrine mechanisms of stress vulnerability and resilience', *Neuropsychopharmacology*, 42 (Jun 2016), pp. 62–80.

45 Ehrlich, K. et al, 'Testing the biological embedding hypothesis: is early life adversity associated with a later proinflammatory phenotype?', *Development and Psychopathology*, 28:4:2 (Nov 2016), pp. 1273–83.

46 Liu, R. et al, 'Socioeconomic status in childhood and C-reactive protein in adulthood: a systematic review and meta-analysis', *Journal of Epidemiology and Community Health*, 71:8 (Feb 2017), pp. 817–26.

47 Moffitt, T. et al, 'A gradient of childhood self-control predicts health, wealth and public safety', *Proceedings of the National Academy of Science USA*, 108:7 (Jan 2011), pp. 2693–8.

48 Marshall, J., 'Children's self-control predicts health, wealth', NBC News (25 Jan 2011).

49 Danese, A. et al, 'Childhood maltreatment predicts adult inflammation in a life-course study', *Proceedings of the National Academy of Sciences USA*, 104:4 (Jan 2007), pp. 1319–24; Danese, A. and Lewis, S., 'Psychoneuroimmunology of early-life stress: the hidden wounds of childhood trauma?', *Neuropsychopharmacology*, 42 (2017), pp. 99–114.

50 Moffitt, T. et al, 'Childhood exposure to violence and lifelong health: clinical intervention science and stress biology research join forces', *Developmental Psychopathology*, 25 (Nov 2013), 4:0:2.

51 Pearson, H., *The Life Project* (Penguin, 2016).

52 Cooper, C., *Guardian* obituary of David Barker (11 September 2013).

Notes

PART TWO

The Body Under Construction

3. Starting with cells

1 Capra, F., *The Hidden Connections* (Flamingo, 2003).
2 Popkin, G., 'Bacteria use brain-like bursts of electricity to communicate', *Quanta, Scientific American* (9 September 2017); Niehoff, D., *The Language of Life* (Joseph Henry Press, 2005).
3 quoted in Blasi, C. et al, 'When development matters: from evolutionary psychology to evolutionary developmental psychology', *Anuario de Psicologia*, 39:2 (Sep 2008), pp. 177–191.
4 Panksepp, J., *Affective Neuroscience: The Foundations of Human and Animal Emotions* (Oxford University Press, 1998).
5 Watt, D., 'In Memoriam: Personal reflections on the neuroscientific legacy of Jaak Panksepp (1943–2017)', *Emotion Researcher*, ISRE, July 2017.
6 Ibid.
7 Stiles, J. and Jernigan, T., 'The basics of brain development', *Neuropsychology Review*, 20:4 (Nov 2010), pp. 327–48.
8 Wolpert, L., *How We Live and Why We Die* (Faber and Faber, 2009).
9 Ackerman, S., *Discovering the Brain* (National Academies Press, 1992).
10 Komaroff, A. and Scripps-Howard News Service, 'Ask Doctor K, learning how cells age may lead to anti-aging treatment', *Times Standard* (30 July 2018).
11 Damasio, A., *Self Comes to Mind* (Vintage Books, 2010).
12 Damasio, A., *The Strange Order of Things: Life, Feeling and the Making of Cultures* (Vintage Books, 2018).
13 Damasio, A., *Self Comes to Mind*.
14 Theise, N., and Harris, R., 'Postmodern biology' in Wobus, A. and Boheler, K. (eds.), *Stem Cells* (Springer Verlag, 2006).
15 Burr, V., *Social Constructionism* (Routledge, 2015).
16 Dennett, D., *Darwin's Dangerous Idea* (Simon & Schuster, 1995).

Notes

4. Growing inside mother's body

1 Napso, T. et al, 'The role of the placental hormones in mediating maternal adaptations to support pregnancy and lactation', *Frontiers in Physiology*, 9 (Aug 2018), article 1091; Hoekzema, E. et al, 'Pregnancy leads to long-lasting changes in human brain structure', *Nature Neuroscience*, 20 (2017); Soma-Pillay, P. et al, 'Physiological changes in pregnancy', *Cardiovascular Journal of Africa*, 27:2 (Mar–Apr 2016), pp. 89–94.
2 Pervolaraki, E. et al, 'Ventricular myocardium development and the role of connexions in the human fetal heart', *Scientific Reports*, 7 (Sep 2017), article 12272.
3 Tau, G. and Petersen, B., 'Normal development of brain circuits', *Neuropsychopharmacology*, 35:1 (2010), pp. 147–68.
4 Edwards, S. et al, 'The maternal gut microbiome during pregnancy', *MCN American Journal of Maternal/Child Nursing*, 42:6 (Nov–Dev 2017), pp. 310–17.
5 Hoekzema, E. et al, 'Becoming a mother entails anatomical changes in the ventral striatum of the human brain that facilitate its responsiveness to offspring cues', *Psychoneuroendocrinology*, 112 (Feb 2020), article 104507.
6 Burton, G. et al, 'Placental origins of chronic disease', *Physiological Review*, 96:4 (Oct 2016), pp. 1509–65.
7 Phillips, A. et al, 'Neonatal iron status is impaired by maternal obesity and excessive weight gain in infancy', *Journal of Perinatology*, 34:7 (Jul 2014), pp. 513–18; Lozoff, B. et al, 'Long-lasting neural and behavioural effects of iron deficiency in infancy', *Nutrition Reviews*, 64:5:2 (May 2006), S34–S91.
8 Palmer, A., 'Nutritionally mediated programming of the developing immune system', *Advances in Nutrition*, 2:5 (Sep 2011), pp. 377–395.
9 Fekete, K. et al, 'Perinatal folate supply: relevance in health outcome parameters', *Maternal and Child Nutrition*, 6:2 (Oct 2010), pp. 23–38; Corstius, H. et al, 'Effect of intrauterine growth restriction on the number of cardiomyocytes in rats', *Pediatric Research*, 57:6 (Jun 2005), pp. 796–800.

10 Painter, R., Roseboom, T. and Bleker, O., 'Prenatal exposure to the Dutch famine and disease in later life: an overview', *Reproductive Toxicology*, 20:3 (Sep–Oct 2005), pp. 345–52; Heijmans, B. et al, 'Persistent epigenetic differences associated with prenatal exposure to famine in humans', *Proceedings of the National Academy of Science USA*, 105:44 (Sep 2008), pp. 17046–17049.

11 Botto, L. et al, 'Lower rate of selected congenital heart defects with better maternal diet quality: a population- based study', *Archives of Disease in Childhood – Fetal and Neonatal Edition*, 101 (Jan 2016), pp. 43–9.

12 Marshall, N. et al, 'The importance of nutrition in pregnancy and lactation: lifelong consequences', *American Journal of Obstetrics and Gynecology*, 226:5 (May 2022), pp. 607–632.

13 Kalisch-Smith, J. et al, 'Environmental risk factors for congenital heart disease', *Cold Spring Harbor Perspectives in Biology*, 12:3 (Mar 2020) a037234.

14 Wood-Bradley, R. et al, 'Understanding the role of maternal diet on kidney development; an opportunity to improve cardiovascular and renal health for future generations', *Nutrients*, 7:3 (Mar 2015), pp. 1881–1905.

15 Entringer, S., 'Impact of stress and stress physiology during pregnancy on child metabolic function and obesity risk', *Current opinion in Clinical Nutrition and Metabolic Care*, 16:3 (May 2013), pp. 320–327; Boehmer, B. et al, 'The impact of IUGR on pancreatic islet development and beta cell function', *Endocrinology*, 235:2 (2017), R63–R76.

16 Barker, D. et al, 'Weight in infancy and death from ischaemic heart disease', *The Lancet*, 2:8663 (Sep 1989), pp. 577–580; Burton, G. et al, 'Placental origins of chronic disease', *Physiological Review*.

17 Boseley, S., 'Junk food diet "stunting Nepalese children's growth"', *Guardian* (17 July 2016).

18 Soderborg, T. et al, 'The gut microbiota in infants of obese mothers increases inflammation and susceptibility to NAFLD', *Nature Communications*, 9 (Oct 2018), article 4462.

19 Segovia, S., 'Maternal obesity, inflammation and developmental programming', *BioMed Research International*, (May 2014), article 41897.

20 Helle, E. and Priest, J., 'Maternal obesity and diabetes mellitus as risk factors for congenital heart disease in the offspring', *Journal of the American Heart Association*, 9:8 (Apr 2020), e011541.

21 Stansfield, B. et al, 'Nonlinear relationship between birthweight and visceral fat in adolescents', *The Journal of Pediatrics*, 174 (2016), pp. 185–92.

22 Hillier, T. et al, 'Childhood obesity and metabolic imprinting', *Diabetes Care*, 30:9 (2007), pp. 2287–92.

23 Ong, Z. and Muhlhausler, B., 'Maternal "junk-food" feeding of rat dams alters food choices and development of the mesolimbic reward pathway in the offspring', *The Journal of the Federation of American Societies for Experimental Biology*, 25:7 (2011), pp. 2167–79.

24 Simopoulos, A., 'An increase in the Omega6/Omega3 fatty acid ratio increases the risk for obesity', *Nutrients*, 8:3 (2016), p. 128; Massiera, F. et al, 'A Western-like fat diet is sufficient to induce a gradual enhancement in fat mass over generations', *Journal of Lipid Research*, 51:8 (2010), pp. 2352–61.

25 Teicholz, N., 'A short history of saturated fat: the making and unmaking of a scientific consensus', *Current Opinion in Endocrinology, Diabetes and Obesity*, 30:1 (Feb 2023), pp. 65–71.

26 Boseley, S., 'Ultra-processed products now half of all UK family food purchases', *Guardian* (2 February 2018).

27 López-Vicente, M. et al, 'Prenatal omega-6: omega-3 ratio and ADHD symptoms', *The Journal of Pediatrics* (Jun 2019).

28 Rundle, A. et al, 'Association of childhood obesity with maternal exposure to ambient air polycyclic aromatic hydrocarbons during pregnancy', *American Journal of Epidemiology*, 175:11 (2012), pp. 1163–72.

29 Kim, D. et al, 'Air pollutants and early origins of respiratory diseases', *Chronic Diseases and Translational Medicine*, 4 (Jun 2018), pp. 75–94.

30 Ailhaud, G. et al, 'Temporal changes in dietary fats: role of n6 PUFAs in excessive adipose tissue development and relationship to obesity', *Progress in Lipid Research*, 45:3 (2006), pp. 203–36; Massiera, F. et al, 'A Western-like fat diet is sufficient to induce a gradual enhancement in

fat mass over generations', *Journal of Lipid Research*; Kabaran, S. and Besler, H. T., 'Do fatty acids affect fetal programming?' *Journal of Health Population and Nutrition*, 33 (Aug 2015), p. 14.

31 Segovia, S., 'Maternal obesity, inflammation and developmental programming'.

32 Spalding, K. et al, 'Dynamics of fat cell turnover in humans', *Nature*, 453 (May 2008), pp. 783–7.

33 Daraki, V. et al, 'Low maternal vitamin D status in pregnancy increases the risk of childhood obesity', *Pediatric Obesity*, 13:8 (Aug 2018), pp. 467–75.

34 Spalding, K. et al, 'Dynamics of fat cell turnover in humans'.

35 Entringer, S. et al, 'Maternal cortisol during pregnancy and infant adiposity: a prospective investigation', *Journal of Clinical Endocrinology and Metabolism*, 102:4 (Apr 2017), pp. 1366–74.

36 Gur, T. et al, 'Prenatal stress disrupts social behaviour, cortical neurobiology and commensal microbes in adult male offspring', *Behaviour and Brain Research*, 359 (2019), pp. 886–94; Chen, H., and Gur, T., 'Intrauterine microbiota: missing or the missing link?', *Trends in Neuroscience*, 42:6 (2019), pp. 402–13.

37 Felitti, V., 'Adverse childhood experiences and adult health', *Academic Pediatrics*, 9:3 (2009), pp. 131–32.

38 Omolaoye, T. et al, 'The mutagenic effect of tobacco smoke on male fertility', *Environmental Science and Pollution Research*, 29:41 (2022), pp. 62055–66.

39 Grubb, S., 'Julia Brown, founder of the FASD Trust, stresses dangers of drinking during pregnancy', *Oxford Mail* (24 October 2017).

40 Bandoli, G. et al, 'Patterns of prenatal alcohol use that predict infant growth and development', *Pediatrics*, 143:2 (2019).

41 Bandoli, G. et al, 'Trajectories of prenatal alcohol exposure and behavioral outcomes: findings from a community-based sample', *Drug and Alcohol Dependence*, 233 (Apr 2022), p. 109351.

42 Gluckman, P. and Hanson, M., *The Fetal Matrix: evolution, development and disease* (Cambridge University Press, 2005).

43 Badrick, E. et al, 'The relationship between smoking status and cortisol secretion', *Journal of Clinical Endocrinology and Metabolism*, 92:3 (2007), pp. 819–24.

44 Haan, E. et al, 'Prenatal smoking, alcohol and caffeine exposure and offspring externalising disorders: a systematic review and meta-analysis', *Addiction* (Apr 2022).

45 Gustavson, K. et al, 'Smoking in pregnancy and child ADHD', *Pediatrics*, 139:2 (2017), e20162509.

46 Zhao, L. et al, 'Parental smoking and the risk of congenital heart defects in offspring: an updated meta-analysis of observational studies', *European Journal of Preventive Cardiology*, 27:12 (Mar 2019), pp. 1–10.

47 Wu, C-C. et al, 'Paternal tobacco smoke correlated to offspring asthma and prenatal epigenetic programming', *Frontiers in Genetics*, 10 (May 2019), p. 471.

48 Maritz, G., and Harding, R., 'Lifelong programming implications of exposure to tobacco smoking and nicotine before and soon after birth', *International Journal of Environmental Research and Public Health*, 8 (2011), pp. 875–98; Tiesler, C. and Heinrich, J., 'Prenatal nicotine exposure and child behaviour problems', *European Child and Adolescent Psychiatry*, 23 (2014), pp. 913–29.

49 Hosseinzadeh, A. et al, 'Nicotine induces neutrophil extracellular traps', *Journal of Leucocyte Biology*, 100:5 (2016), p. 1105.

50 Zong, D. et al, 'The role of cigarette smoke-induced epigenetic alterations in inflammation', *Epigenetics and Chromatin*, 12:65 (2019); Wu, C-C. et al, 'Paternal tobacco smoke correlated to offspring asthma and prenatal epigenetic programming'.

51 Winett, L. et al, 'A framework to address challenges in communicating the developmental origins of health and disease', *Current Environmental Health Reports*, 3:3 (2016), pp. 169–77.

52 Armstrong, E., 'Making sense of advice about drinking during pregnancy: does evidence even matter?', *Journal of Perinatal Education*, 26:2 (2017).

53 Sandman, C. et al, 'Fetal exposure to maternal depressive symptoms is associated with cortical thickness in late childhood', *Biological*

Psychiatry, 77:4 (2015), pp. 324–34; Davis, E. et al, 'Prenatal maternal stress, child cortical thickness and adolescent depressive symptoms', *Child Development* (2019); Buss, C. et al, 'Maternal cortisol over the course of pregnancy and subsequent child amygdala and hippocampus volumes and affective problems', *PNAS USA*, 109: 20 (2012), E1312–19.

54 Thornburg, K. and Marshall, N., 'The placenta is the center of the chronic disease universe', *American Journal of Obstetrics and Gynaecology*, 213:40 (2015), S14–S20.

55 Roth, G. et al, 'Global burden of CVD and risk factors 1990-2019: update for the Global Burden of Disease 2019 study', *Journal of American College of Cardiology*, 76:25 (2020), pp. 2982–3021.

56 Baker, C., 'Obesity Statistics: research briefing', House of Commons Library, UK Parliament, 2023; Trust for America's Health, 2023.

57 Gallagher, J., 'Diabetes cases soar by 60% in past decade', *BBC News* (17 August 2015).

58 Freedom of Information request to NHS England, March 2022 (ref 2203 1715614).

5. The post-natal cocoon

1 Blackburn, V., 'Breast-feeding in public? Just don't do it', *Daily Express* (23 August 2018).

2 Johnson, S. et al, 'The science of early life toxic stress for paediatric practice and advocacy', *Pediatrics*, 131:2 (2013), pp. 319–27.

3 Sendak, M., *In the Night Kitchen* (Harper and Row, 1970).

4 Riskin, A. et al, 'Changes in immunomodulatory constituents of human milk in response to active infection in the nursing infant', *Pediatric Research*, 71:2 (2012), pp. 220–5.

5 Sender, R. et al, 'Revised estimates for the number of human and bacteria cells in the body', *PLOS Biology*, 14:8 (2016), e1002533.

6 Liu, W. et al, 'Alteration of behaviour and monoamine levels attributed to *lactobacillus plantarum* PS128 in germ-free mice', *Behavioural Brain Research*, 298:part B (2016), pp. 202–9; Mayer, E. et al, 'Gut microbes

and the brain: paradigm shift in neuroscience', *Journal of Neuroscience*, 34:46 (2014), pp. 15490–96.
7   Zhang, N. et al, 'Efficacy of probiotics on stress in healthy volunteers: a systematic review and meta-analysis based on randomised controlled trials', *Brain and Behaviour*, 10:9 (2020).
8   Parnanen, K. et al, 'Early-life formula feeding is associated with infant gut microbiota alterations and an increased antibiotic resistance load', *American Journal of Clinical Nutrition*, 115:2 (2021), pp. 407–21; Ho, N. et al, 'Meta-analysis of effects of exclusive breastfeeding on infant gut microbiota across generations', *Nature Communications*, 9:1 (2018), p. 4169; Mackie, R. et al, 'Developmental microbial ecology of the neonatal gastrointestinal tract', *The American Journal of Clinical Nutrition*, 69:5 (1999), pp. 1035–45; Guaraldi, F. and Salvatori, G., 'Effect of breast and formula feeding on gut microbiota shaping in newborns', *Frontiers in Cellular and Infection Microbiology*, 2:94 (2012).
9   O'Sullivan, A. et al, 'The influence of early infant-feeding practices on the intestinal microbiome and body composition in infants', *Nutrition and Metabolic Insights*, 8:1 (2015), p. 87.
10 Gibbering Ginger, 2 Mar 2010, 13:30:23.
11 UNICEF UK, 'Breastfeeding in the UK', 2018.
12 Borewicz, K. et al, 'The effect of prebiotic fortified infant formulas on microbiota composition and dynamics in early life', *Scientific Reports*, 9 (2019), article 2434.
13 Buhrer, C. et al, 'Infant formulas with synthetic oligosaccharides and respective marketing practices', *Molecular and Cellular Pediatrics*, 9:14 (2022); Laursen, M., 'Gut microbiota development: influence of diet from infancy to toddlerhood', *Annals of Nutrition and Metabolism*, 77 (2021), pp. 21–34.
14 Clarke, G. et al, 'Gut reactions: breaking down xenobiotic-microbiome interactions', *Pharmacological Review*, 71 (2019), pp. 198–224; Meng, C. et al, 'Human gut microbiota and gastrointestinal cancer', *Genomics Proteomics Bioinformatics*, 16 (2018), pp. 33–49; Zhu, Q. et al, 'Dysbiosis signatures of gut microbiota in coronary

artery disease', *Physiological Genomics*, 50 (2018), pp. 893–903; Gazerani, P., 'Probiotics for Parkinson's Disease', *International Journal of Molecular Sciences* 20:17 (Aug 2019), p. 4121.

15 Lyon, L., '"All disease begins in the gut": was Hippocrates right?', *Brain*, 141:3 (Feb 2018), pp. 1–5; Mueller, N. et al, 'The infant microbiome development: mom matters', *Trends in Molecular Medicine*, 21:2 (2015), pp. 109–117; Thursby, E. and Juge, N., 'Introduction to the human gut microbiota', *Biochemical Journal*, 474 (2017), pp. 1823–36.

16 Dinan, T. and Cryan, J., 'Gut instincts: microbiota as a key regulator of brain development, ageing and neurodegeneration', *The Journal of Physiology*, 595:2 (2017), pp. 489–503.

17 Damasio, A., *The Strange Order of Things*.

18 Francino, P., 'Early development of the gut microbiota and human health', *Pathogens*, 4 (2014), pp. 769–90.

19 Belkaid, Y. and Hand, T., 'Role of the microbiota in immunity and inflammation', *Cell*, 157:1 (2014), pp. 121–41.

20 Pradeu, T., 'A mixed self: the role of symbiosis in development', *Biological Theory*, 6:1 (2011), pp. 80–88.

21 Dinan, T. et al, 'Collective unconscious: how gut microbes shape human behaviour', *Journal of Psychiatric Research*, 63 (2015), pp. 1–9; Farzi, A. et al, 'Gut microbiota and the neuroendocrine system', *Neurotherapeutics*, 15:1 (2018), pp. 5–22.

22 Baumeister, D. et al, 'Childhood trauma and adulthood inflammation: a meta-analysis of peripheral CRP, IL-6 and TNF-alpha', *Molecular Psychiatry*, 21 (2016), pp. 642–49; Puig, J. et al, 'Predicting adult physical illness from infant attachment: a prospective longitudinal study', *Health Psychology*, 32:4 (2013), pp. 409–17; Lewis, C. et al, 'Epigenetic differences in inflammation genes of monozygotic twins are related to parent-child emotional availability and health', *Brain, Behaviour and Immunity, Health*, 5 (May 2020), 100084.

23 Lewis, C. et al, 'Epigenetic differences in inflammation genes of monozygotic twins are related to parent-child emotional availability and health'.

24 Koenig, W., 'CRP: a sensitive marker of inflammation predicts future risk of coronary heart disease', *Circulation*, 99 (1999), pp. 237–42.
25 McDade, T. et al, 'Long-term effects of birth weight and breastfeeding duration on inflammation in early adulthood', *Proceedings. Biological Sciences*, 281:1784 (Apr 2014), 20133116; Ridker, P. et al, 'Rosuvastatin to prevent vascular events in men and women with elevated c-reactive protein', *New England Journal of Medicine*, 359 (2008), pp. 2195–2207.
26 Dubois, N. and Gregory, K., 'Characterizing the intestinal microbiome in infantile colic: findings based on an integrative review of the literature', *Biological Research for Nursing*, 18:3 (May 2016), pp. 307–15; Rhoads, M. et al, 'Infant colic represents inflammation and dysbiosis', *Journal of Pediatrics*, 203 (2018), pp. 55–61.
27 Georgountzou, A. and Papadopoulos, N., 'Postnatal innate immune development: from birth to adulthood', *Frontiers in Immunology*, 8 (2017), p. 957.
28 Belkaid, Y. and Hand, T., 'Role of the microbiota in immunity and inflammation'; Maddux, A. and Douglas, I., 'Is the developmentally immature immune response in paediatric sepsis a recapitulation of immune tolerance?', *Immunology*, 145 (2015), pp. 1–10; Schmiedeberg, K. et al, 'T cells of infants are mature, but hypo-reactive due to limited Ca_{2+} influx', *PloS One*, 11:11 (2016), e0166633.
29 Schaffert, S. and Khatri, P., 'Early life immunity in the era of systems biology: understanding development and disease', *Genome Medicine*, 10:88 (2018).
30 Baban, B. et al, 'Presence and profile of innate lymphoid cells in human breast milk', *JAMA Pediatrics*, 172:6 (2018), pp. 594–96.
31 Ardeshir, A. et al, 'Breast-fed and bottle-fed infant rhesus macaques develop distinct gut microbiotas and immune systems', *Science Translational Medicine*, 6:252 (Sep 2014).
32 Mulligan, C. and Friedman, J., 'Maternal modifiers of the infant gut microbiota-metabolic consequences', *Journal of Endocrinology*, 235:1 (Oct 2017), R1–R12.
33 Hsu, P., and Nanan, R., 'Does breast milk nurture T lymphocytes in their cradle?', *Frontiers in Pediatrics*, 6 (2018), article 268; Hasselbalch, H.

et al, 'Decreased thymus size in formula-fed infants compared with breast-fed infants', *Acta Paediatrica*, 85 (1996), pp. 1029–32.

34 Wood, H. et al, 'Breastfeeding promotes early neonatal regulatory T-cell expansion and immune tolerance of non-inherited maternal antigens', *Allergy*, 76:8 (2021), pp. 2447–60.

35 Jakaitis, B. and Denning, P., 'Human breast milk and the gastrointestinal innate immune system', *Clinical Perinatology*, 41:2 (2014), pp. 423–35; Victora, C., quoted in UNICEF Baby Friendly Initiative press release, 'The Lancet: increasing breast feeding worldwide could prevent over 800,000 child deaths every year' (2016).

36 Victora, C. et al, 'Breastfeeding in the 21st century: epidemiology, mechanisms and lifelong effect', *The Lancet* 387 (2016), pp. 475–90.

37 Martens, P. et al, 'Breastfeeding helps to prevent type 1 diabetes', *Diabetes Care* (May 2017); dc170016. https://doi.org/10.2337/dc17-0016.

38 Su, Q. et al, 'Breastfeeding and the risk of childhood cancer: a systematic review and dose-response meta-analysis', *BMC Medicine*, 19:90 (2021).

39 Wang, X. et al, 'Breastfeeding in infancy and mortality in middle and late adulthood: a prospective cohort study and meta-analysis', *Journal of Internal Medicine*, 293 (2023), pp. 624–35.

40 Adab, P. et al, 'Breastfeeding practice, oral contraceptive use, and risk of rheumatoid arthritis amongst Chinese women: the Guanzhou Biobank Cohort Study', *Rheumatology*, 53:5 (May 2014), pp. 860–6.

41 Su, D. et al, 'Ovarian cancer risk is reduced by prolonged lactation: a case-control study in southern China', *The American Journal of Clinical Nutrition*, 97:2 (2013), pp. 354–59.

42 Tschiderer, L. et al, 'Breastfeeding is associated with a reduced maternal cardiovascular risk: systematic review and meta-analysis', *Journal of the American Heart Association*, 11 (2022), e022746.

43 Shields, B., *Down Came the Rain* (Hyperion, 2005).

44 'BBC DJ Alex Dyke suspended over breastfeeding remarks', BBC News (13 August 2015).

45 Oakley, L. et al, 'Factors associated with breastfeeding in England: an analysis by primary care trust', *BMJ Open* (2013).

46 Swami, V. et al, 'The Breast Size Satisfaction Survey: Breast size dissatisfaction and its antecedents and outcomes in women from 40 nations', *Body Image*, 32 (Feb 2020), pp. 199–217.
47 Ibid.
48 Morley-Hewitt, A. and Owen, A., 'A systematic review examining the association between female body image and the intention, initiation and duration of post-partum feeding methods', *Journal of Health Psychology*, 25:2 (2020), pp. 207–26.
49 UNICEF, 'Breastfeeding in the UK', 2018.
50 Facts and Factors, 'Infant Formula Market by Type (Standard, Follow-on, Toddler, and Specialty) and By Distribution Channel (Hypermarkets/Supermarkets, Pharmacy/Medical Stores, Specialty Stores, and Others): Global Industry Outlook, Market Size, Business Intelligence, Consumer Preferences, Statistical Surveys, Comprehensive Analysis, Historical Developments, Current Trends, and Forecasts, 2020–2026', *Globe Newswire* (January 2021).
51 Baby Milk Action, 2020.
52 Rollins, N. et al, 'Marketing of commercial milk formula: a system to capture parents, communities, science and policy', *The Lancet*, 401 (Feb 2023), pp. 486–502.
53 Rollins, N. et al, 'Breastfeeding 2: Why invest, and what will it take to improve breastfeeding practices?', *The Lancet*, 387 (Jan 2016), pp. 491–504.
54 Cannon, E., 'Breast isn't always best and we have to stop bashing mothers who choose the bottle', *Mail Online* (28 July 2018).
55 van Tulleken, C., *Ultra-Processed People: Why Do We All Eat Stuff That Isn't Food . . . and Why Can't We Stop?* (Cornerstone Press, 2023).
56 Maté, G., *The Myth of Normal* (Vermilion, 2022).
57 Vittner, D. et al, 'Increase in oxytocin from skin-to-skin contact enhances development of parent–infant relationship', *Biological Research for Nursing*, 20:1 (2018), pp. 54–62.
58 Nishizato, M. et al, 'Developmental changes in social attention and oxytocin levels in infants and children', *Scientific Reports*, 7 (May 2017), article 2540.

59 Feldman, R., 'Sensitive periods in human social development: new insights from research on oxytocin, synchrony, and high-risk parenting', *Development and Psychopathology*, 27 (2015), pp. 369–95; Carter, S., 'Oxytocin pathways and the evolution of human behaviour', *Annual Review of Psychology*, 65 (2014), pp. 17–39.

60 Domes, G. et al, 'Oxytocin attenuates amygdala responses to emotional faces regardless of valence', *Biological Psychiatry*, 62 (2007), pp. 1187–90; Colonnello, V. et al, 'Positive social interactions in a lifespan perspective with a focus on opioidergic and oxytocinergic systems: implications for neuroprotection', *Current Neuropharmacology*, 15:4 (2017), pp. 543–61.

61 Clodi, M., 'Oxytocin alleviates the neuroendocrine and cytokine response to bacterial endotoxins in healthy men', *American Journal of Physiology Endocrinology and Metabolism*, 295:3 (2008).

62 Mohiyeddini, C., 'Emotional suppression explains the link between early life stress and plasma oxytocin', *Anxiety Stress Coping*, 27:4 (2014), pp. 466–75.

63 Colonnello, V. et al, 'Positive social interactions in a lifespan perspective with a focus on opioidergic and oxytocinergic systems: implications for neuroprotection'.

64 Ellis, B. et al, 'Developmental programming of oxytocin through variation in early-life stress: four meta-analyses and a theoretical re-interpretation', *Clinical Psychology Review*, vol. 86 (2021), article 101985; Feldman, R. et al, 'Parental oxytocin and early caregiving jointly shape children's oxytocin response and social reciprocity', *Neuropsychopharmacology*, 38 (2013), pp. 1154–62; Toepfer, P. et al, 'A role of oxytocin receptor gene brain tissue expression quantitative trait locus rs237895 in the intergenerational transmission of the effects of maternal child maltreatment', *Journal of the American Academy of Child and Adolescent Psychiatry*, 58:12 (2019), pp. 1207–16; Strathearn, L., 'Maternal neglect: oxytocin, dopamine and the neurobiology of attachment', *Neuroendocrinology*, 23 (2011), pp. 1054–65.

65 Ein-Dor, T. et al, 'Epigenetic modification of oxytocin and glucocorticoid receptor genes linked to attachment avoidance in young adults', *Attachment and Human Development*, 20:4 (2018).

66 Borghi, C. and Cicero, A., 'Recent evidence of the role of omega 3 PUFAs on blood pressure control and hypertension-related complications', *Future Lipidology*, 1:5 (2006), pp. 569–77; Begg, A. et al, 'Omega3 fatty acids in cardiovascular disease: re-assessing the evidence', *British Journal of Cardiology*, 19 (2012), pp. 79–84.

67 Begg, D. et al, 'Hypertension induced by omega-3 polyunsaturated fatty acid deficiency is alleviated by alpha-linoleic acid regardless of dietary source', *Hypertension Research*, 33 (2010), pp. 808–13; Weisinger, H. et al, 'Perinatal omega 3 fatty acid deficiency affects blood pressure in later life', *Nature Medicine*, 7:3 (2001).

68 de la Presa Owens, S. and Innes, S., 'DHA and arachidonic acid prevent a decrease in dopamine and serotonin neurotransmitters in frontal cortex', *Journal of Nutrition*, 129 (1999), pp. 2088–93; Kodas, E., 'Serotoninergic neurotransmission is affected by n-3 polyunsaturated fatty acids in the rat', *Journal of Neurochemistry*, 89 (2004), pp. 695–402; Sublette, E. et al, 'PUFA associates with dopaminergic indices in major depressive disorder', *International Journal of Neuropsychopharmacology*, 17:3 (2014), pp. 383–91; Patrick, R. and Ames, B., 'Vitamin D and Omega 3 fatty acids control serotonin synthesis and action', *FASEB Journal*, 29:6 (2015), pp. 2205–2679.

69 Healy-Stoffel, M. and Levant, B., 'N3 (Omega3) fatty acids: effects on brain dopamine systems and potential role in the etiology of neuropsychiatric disorders', *Central Nervous System Neurological Disorders: Drug Targets*, 17:3 (2018), pp. 216–32.

70 Laye, S. et al, 'Anti-inflammatory effects of omega-3 fatty acids in the brain: physiological mechanisms and relevance to pharmacology', *Pharmacological Reviews*, 70:1 (2018) pp. 12–38; McNamara, R. et al, 'Omega 3 fatty acid deficiency increases constitutive pro-inflammatory cytokine production in rats: relationship with central serotonin turnover', *Prostaglandins Leukotrienes Essential Fatty Acids*, 83:4–6 (2010), pp. 185–91; Madore, C. et al, 'Nutritional n-3 PUFAs deficiency during perinatal periods alters brain innate immune system and neuronal plasticity-associated genes', *Brain, Behaviour and Immunity*, 41 (2014), pp. 22–31.

71 Kodas, E. et al, 'Reversibility of n-3 fatty acid deficiency-induced changes in dopaminergic neurotransmission in rats: critical role of developmental stage', *Journal of Lipid Research*, 43 (2022), p. 1209.

72 Serhan, C. et al, 'The resolution code of acute inflammation: novel pro-resolving lipid mediators in resolution', *Seminars in Immunology*, 27:3 (2015), pp. 200–215; Calder, P., 'n-3 PUFAs, inflammation and inflammatory diseases', *The American Journal of Clinical Nutrition*, 83:6 (2006), 1505S–1519S.

73 Carhart-Harris, R. and Nutt, D., 'Serotonin and brain function: a tale of two receptors', *Journal of Psychopharmacology*, 31:9 (2017), pp. 1091–1120.

74 Chang, C. et al, 'Abnormal serotonin transporter availability in the brains of adults with conduct disorder', *Journal of the Formosan Medical Association*, 116 (2017), pp. 469–75; aan hen Rot, M. et al, 'Social behaviour and mood in everyday life: the effects of tryptophan in quarrelsome individuals', *Journal of Psychiatry and Neuroscience*, 31:4 (2006), pp. 253–62.

75 Lambe, E. et al, 'Serotonin receptor expression in human prefrontal cortex', *PLoS One*, 6:7 (2011), e22799.

76 Suomi, S. et al, 'Reactivity and behavioural inhibition as personality traits in non-human primates', in Weiss, A., and King, J. (eds), *Personality and Temperament in Non-human Primates*, (Springer, 2011).

77 Kinnally, E. et al, 'Effects of early experience and genotype on serotonin transporter regulation in infant rhesus macaques', *Genes, Brain and Behaviour*, 7 (2008), pp. 481–86.

78 Shannon, C. et al, 'Maternal absence and stability of individual differences in CSF 5-HIAA concentrations in rhesus monkey infants', *American Journal of Psychiatry*, 162 (2005), pp. 1158–64.

79 Suomi, S. et al, 'Reactivity and behavioural inhibition as personality traits in non-human primates'.

80 Miller, J. et al, 'Reported childhood abuse is associated with low serotonin transporter binding in vivo in major depressive disorder', *Synapse*, 63:7 (2009), pp. 565–73.

81 Maurer-Spurej, E. et al, 'Platelet serotonin levels support depression scores for women with postpartum depression', *Journal of Psychiatry and Neuroscience*, 32:1 (2007), pp. 23–29.

82 Moncrieff, J. et al, 'The serotonin theory of depression: a systematic umbrella review of the evidence', *Molecular Psychiatry*, 28 (2022), pp. 3243–56.

83 Martin, C. et al, 'The Brain-Gut-Microbiome Axis', *Cellular and Molecular Gastroenterology and Hepatology*, 6:2 (2018), pp. 133–1148.

84 Chen, Y. et al, 'Regulation of neurotransmitters by the gut microbiota and effects on cognition in neurological disorders', *Nutrients*, 13:6 (2021), p. 2099; O'Mahony, S. et al, 'Serotonin, tryptophan metabolism and the brain-gut-microbiome axis', *Behaviour and Brain Research*, 277 (2015), pp. 32–48; Yano, J. et al, 'Indigenous bacteria from the gut microbiota regulate host serotonin biosynthesis', *Cell*, 161:2 (2015), pp. 264–76.

85 Nguyen, T. et al, 'Coupling between prefrontal brain activity and respiratory sinus arrhythmia in infants and adults', *Developmental Cognitive Neuroscience*, 53 (2022), 101047.

86 Neuhuber, W. and Berthoud, H.-R., 'Functional anatomy of the vagus system: how does the polyvagal theory comply?', *Biological Psychology*, 174 (Oct 2022).

87 Colonnello, V. et al, 'Positive social interactions in a lifespan perspective with a focus on opioidergic and oxytocinergic systems: implications for neuroprotection', *Current Neuropharmacology*, 15 (2017), pp. 543–61.

88 Porges, S. and Furman, E., 'The early development of the autonomic nervous system provides a neural platform for social behaviour: a polyvagal perspective'; Feldman, R. et al, 'Mother and infant coordinate heart rhythms through episodes of interaction synchrony', *Infant Behavior and Development*, 34:4 (2011), pp. 569–77.

89 Abney, D. et al, 'Associations between infant-mother physiological synchrony and 4- to 6-month-old infants' emotion regulation', *Developmental Psychobiology*, (July 2021).

90 Huffman, L. et al, 'Infant temperament and cardiac vagal tone: assessments at 12 weeks of age', *Child Development*, 69:3 (1998), pp. 624–35; Field, T. and Diego, M., 'Vagal activity, early growth and emotional development', *Infant Behaviour and Development*, 31:3 (2008), pp. 261–373.

91 Feldman, R., 'Sensitive periods in human social development: new insights from research on oxytocin, synchrony, and high-risk parenting'.

92 Diamond, L. et al, 'Attachment style, vagal tone and empathy during mother-adolescent interactions', *Journal of Research on Adolescence*, 22:1 (2011), pp. 165–84.

93 Kok, B. et al, 'How positive emotions build physical health: perceived positive social connections account for the upward spiral between positive emotions and vagal tone', *Psychological Science*, (May 2013); Koopman, F. et al, 'Vagus nerve stimulation inhibits cytokine production and attenuates disease severity in rheumatoid arthritis', *PNAS*, 113:29 (2016), pp. 8284–89.

94 Matteoli, G. and Boeckxstaens, G., 'The vagal innervation of the gut and immune homeostasis', *Gut*, 62 (2013), pp. 1214–22.

95 Castanon, L., 'These bacteria may be the key to treating clinical depression', *Medicalxpress*, (2018).

96 Knox, J., *Self-Agency in Psychotherapy* (W.W. Norton & Co, 2011).

97 Graziano, P. et al, 'Maternal behaviour and children's early emotion regulation skills differentially predict development of children's reactive control and later effortful control', *Infant and Child Development*, 19:4 (Jul 2010), pp. 333–53.

98 Gerhardt, S., *Why Love Matters: How Affection Shapes a Baby's Brain* (Routledge, 2014).

99 Porges, S., Bulletproof blog, episode 264.

Notes

PART THREE

When Things Go Wrong

6. Unprotected: stressful relationships and how they affect health

1 Jay, A. et al, 'The Report of the Independent Inquiry into Child Sexual Abuse, House of Commons', 720, 2022.
2 Kellaway, K., 'Sharon Olds: "I want a poem to be useful" ', *Observer* (6 January 2013).
3 Stevens, J., 'The ACE Study – the largest, most important health study you've never heard about', *ACEs Too High News* blog (ACESTOOHIGH.COM), 2012.
4 Nakazawa, D., *Childhood Disrupted* (Simon & Schuster, 2015).
5 Couper, S. and Mackie, P., 'Polishing the Diamonds: addressing ACEs in Scotland', ScotPHN Report, 2016.
6 Kelly-Irving, M. et al, 'Childhood adversity as a risk for cancer: findings from the 1958 British birth cohort survey', *BioMedCentral Public Health*, 13:767 (2013).
7 Hashemi, L. et al, 'Exploring the health burden of cumulative and specific adverse childhood experiences in New Zealand: results from a population-based study', *Child Abuse and Neglect*, 122 (2021), article 105372; Hughes, K. et al, 'The effect of multiple adverse childhood experiences on health: a systematic review and meta-analysis', *Lancet Public Health*, 2 (2017), e356–66.
8 Felitti, V., 'Adverse childhood experiences and adult health'; Felitti, V. and Anda, R., 'The relationship of adverse childhood experiences to adult health, well-being, social function and healthcare', in Lanius, Vermetten and Pain (eds.), *The Impact of Early Life Trauma on Health and Disease: The Hidden Epidemic* (Cambridge University Press, 2010).
9 Gay, R., *Hunger* (Little, Brown Book Group, 2018).
10 Brewer-Smyth, K. et al, 'Childhood adversity and mental health correlates of obesity in a population at risk', *Journal of Correctional Health Care*, 22:4 (2016), pp. 367–382.

11 Barboza Solis, C. et al, 'Adverse childhood experiences and physiological wear and tear in midlife: Findings from the 1958 British birth cohort', *PNAS USA*, 112:7 (2015).

12 Keiley, M. et al, 'The timing of child physical maltreatment: a cross-domain growth analysis of impact on adolescent externalising and internalising problems', *Developmental Psychopathology*, 13:4 (2001), pp. 891–912.

13 Dunn, E. et al, 'Is developmental timing of trauma exposure associated with depressive and PTSD symptoms in adulthood?', *Journal of Psychiatric Research*, 84 (2017), pp. 119–27.

14 Kaplow, J. and Widom, C., 'Age of onset of child maltreatment predicts long-term mental health outcomes', *Journal of Abnormal Psychology*, 116:1 (2007), pp. 176–87.

15 Hambrick, E. et al, 'Beyond the ACE score: examining relationships between timing of developmental adversity, relational health and developmental outcomes in children', *Archives of Psychiatric Nursing*, 33:3 (2019), pp. 238–47.

16 Moore, G., 'Parent conflict predicts infants' vagal regulation in social interaction', *Development and Psychopathology*, 22:1 (2010), pp. 23–33; Porter, C. and Dyer, J., 'Does marital conflict predict infants' physiological regulation? A short-term prospective study', *Journal of Family Psychology*, 31:4 (2017), pp. 475–84.

17 Widom, C. et al, 'A prospective investigation of physical health outcomes in abused and neglected children: new findings from a 30-year follow-up', *American Journal of Public Health*, 102:6 (2012).

18 Lundgren, M. et al, 'Influence of early-life parental severe life events on the risk of type 1 diabetes in children: the DiPiS study', *Acta Diabetologica*, 55 (2018), pp. 797–804; Nygren, M. et al, 'Experience of a serious life event increases the risk for childhood type 1 diabetes: the ABIS population-based prospective cohort study', *Diabetologia* 58 (2015), pp. 1188–97.

19 Bengtsson, J. et al, 'Accumulation of childhood adversities and type 1 diabetes risk: a register-based cohort study of all children born in Denmark between 1980 and 2015', *International Journal of Epidemiology*, 49:5 (2020), pp. 1604–13.

20 Kaleycheva, N. et al, 'The role of lifetime stressors in adult fibromyalgia: systematic review and meta-analysis of case-control studies', *Psychological Medicine*, 51 (2021), pp. 177–93; Parrish, C. et al, 'Childhood adversity and adult onset of hypertension and heart disease in Sao Paulo, Brazil', *Preventing Chronic Disease*, 10 (2013), article 130193; Lei, M.-K. et al, 'Childhood adversity and cardiovascular disease risk: an appraisal of recall methods with a focus on stress-buffering processes in childhood and adulthood', *Social Science & Medicine*, 246 (2020), p. 112794.

21 Repetti, R. et al, 'Allostatic processes in the family', *Development and Psychopathology*, 23:3 (2011), pp. 921–38.

22 Widom, C. et al, 'A prospective investigation of physical health outcomes in abused and neglected children'; Boeck, C. et al, 'Inflammation in adult women with a history of child maltreatment: the involvement of mitochondrial alterations and oxidative stress', *Mitochondrion*, 30: (2016), pp. 197–207; Carlsson, E. et al, 'Psychological stress in children may alter the immune response', *Journal of Immunology*, 192:5 (2014), pp. 2071–81.

23 Repetti, R. et al, 'Allostatic processes in the family'.

24 Ehrlich, K. et al, 'Testing the biological embedding hypothesis: is early life adversity associated with a later proinflammatory phenotype?'

25 Cohen, S. et al, 'Chronic stress, glucocorticoid receptor resistance, inflammation and disease risk', *PNAS*, 109:16 (2012), pp. 5995–99.

26 Coelho, R. et al, 'Childhood maltreatment and inflammatory markers: a systematic review', *Acta Psychiatrica Scandinavica*, (2013), pp. 1–13; Carpenter, L. et al, 'Association between plasma IL-6 response to acute stress and early-life adversity in healthy adults', *Neuropsychopharmacology*, 35 (2010), pp. 2617–23; Liu, R. et al, 'Socioeconomic status in childhood and C-reactive protein in adulthood: a systematic review and meta-analysis'; Avitsur, R. et al, 'Role of early stress in the individual differences in host response to viral infection', *Brain Behaviour and Immunity*, 20:4 (2006), pp. 339–48.

27 Ferrucci, L. and Fabbri, E., 'Inflammageing: chronic inflammation in ageing, cardiovascular disease and frailty', *Nature Reviews Cardiology*, 15:9 (2018), pp. 505–22.

Notes

28 Kiecolt-Glaser, J. et al, 'Close relationships, inflammation and health', *Neuroscience and Biobehavioral Reviews*, 35:1 (2010), pp. 33–38; Nusslock, R. and Miller, G., 'Early-life adversity and physical and mental health across the lifespan: a neuroimmune network hypothesis', *Biological Psychiatry*, 80:1 (2016), pp. 23–32.

29 Pham-Huy, L. et al, 'Free radicals, antioxidants in disease and health', *International Journal of Biomedical Science*, 4:2 (2008).

30 Biswas, S., 'Does the interdependence between oxidative stress and inflammation explain the antioxidant paradox?', *Oxidative Medicine and Cellular Longevity*, (2016), article 5698931; Teodoro, J. et al, 'Therapeutic options targeting oxidative stress, mitochondrial dysfunction and inflammation to hinder the progression of vascular complications of diabetes', *Frontiers in Physiology*, 9 (2019), article 1857.

31 Recchiuti, A. and Serhan, C., 'Pro-resolving lipid mediators (SPMs) and their actions in regulating miRNA in novel resolution circuits in inflammation', *Frontiers in Immunology*, 3:298 (2012); Serhan, C. et al, 'The resolution code of acute inflammation: novel pro-resolving lipid mediators in resolution', *Seminars in Immunology*, 27:3 (2015), pp. 200–15; Fredman, G. and Tabas, I., 'Boosting inflammation resolution in atherosclerosis: the next frontier for therapy', *American Journal of Pathology*, 187:6 (2017), pp. 1211–22; Joffre, C. et al, 'n3 polyunsaturated fatty acids and their derivates reduce neuroinflammation during ageing', *Nutrients*, 12:3 (2020), p. 647.

32 Levy, B., 'Resolvin D1 and Resolvin E1 promote the resolution of allergic airway inflammation', *Frontiers in Immunology*, 3 (2012), article 390.

33 López-Vicario, C. et al, 'Leukocytes from obese individuals exhibit an impaired SPM signature', *FASEB Journal*, 33:6 (Jun 2019), pp. 7072–7083.

34 Marcum, Z. and Hanlon, J., 'Recognizing the risk of chronic nonsteroidal anti-inflammatory drug use in older adults', *The Annals of Long-term Care*, 18:9 (2010), pp. 24–27; Wongrakpanich, S. et al, 'A comprehensive review of NSAID use in the elderly', *Aging and Disease*, 9:1 (2018), pp. 143–50.

35 Chamani, S., Bianoni, V. et al, 'Resolution of inflammation in neurodegenerative diseases: the role of resolvins', *Mediators of Inflammation* (2020), article 3267172; Sochocka, M. et al, 'The gut microbiome alterations and inflammation-driven pathogenesis of Alzheimer's disease – a critical review', *Molecular Neurobiology* (2018), pp. 1–11.

36 Healy-Stoffel, M. and Levant, B., 'N3 (Omega3) fatty acids: effects on brain dopamine systems and potential role in the etiology of neuropsychiatric disorders'.

37 Davis, M. et al, 'Chronic stress and regulation of cellular markers of inflammation in rheumatoid arthritis: implications for fatigue', *Brain, Behaviour and Immunity*, 22:1 (2008), pp. 24–32.

38 Osimo, E. et al, 'Inflammatory markers in depression: a meta-analysis of mean differences and variability in 5,166 patients and 5,083 controls', *Brain, Behavior and Immunity*, 87 (2020), pp. 901–909; World Health Organization (WHO), 2020, Fact Sheet on Depression.

39 Kiecolt-Glaser, J. et al, 'Close relationships, inflammation and health'.

40 Kohler-Forsberg, O. et al, 'Efficacy of anti-inflammatory treatment on major depressive disorder or depressive symptoms: meta-analysis of clinical trials', *Acta Psychiatrica Scandinavica*, 139:5 (2019), pp. 404–19.

41 Hantsoo, L. and Zemel, B., 'Stress gets into the belly: early life stress and the gut microbiome', *Behavioural Brain Research*, 414 (20210), article 113474.

42 Madan, S. and Mehra, M., 'Gut dysbiosis and heart failure: navigating the universe within', *European Journal of Heart Failure*, 22:4 (2020), pp. 629–37.

43 Gagniere, J. et al, 'Gut microbiota imbalance and colorectal cancer', *World Journal of Gastroenterology*, 22:2 (2016), pp. 501–18.

44 Menni, C. et al, ' Gut microbial diversity is associated with lower arterial stiffness in women', *European Heart Journal*, 39:25 (2018), pp. 2390–97.

45 Toya, T. et al, 'Coronary artery disease is associated with an altered gut microbiome composition', *PLoS ONE*, 15:1 (2020), e0227147.

46 Schultess, J. et al, 'The short chain fatty acid Butyrate imprints an antimicrobial program in macrophages', *Immunity*, 50 (2019), pp. 432–445.

47 Herath, M. et al, 'The role of the gastrointestinal mucus system in intestinal homeostasis: implications for neurological disorders', *Frontiers in Cellular and Infection Microbiology* (May 2020).

48 DeJong, E. et al, 'The gut microbiota and unhealthy aging: disentangling cause from consequence', *Cell Host and Microbe*, 28:2 (2020), pp. 180–89.

49 Furman, D. et al, 'Chronic inflammation in the etiology of disease across the life span', *Nature Medicine*, 25 (2019), pp. 1822–32.

50 Rea, I. et al, 'Age and age-related diseases: role of inflammation triggers and cytokines', *Frontiers in Immunology*, 9 (2018); Kiecolt-Glaser, J. et al, 'Childhood adversity heightens the impact of later-life caregiving stress on telomere length and inflammation'; Lu, H. et al, 'Inflammation, a key event in cancer development', *Molecular Cancer Research*, 4:4 (2006).

51 Daneshkhar, A. et al, 'The possible role of vitamin D in suppressing cytokine storm and associated mortality in COVID-19 patients', *medRxiv* (not peer reviewed) (18 May 2020).

52 Esmon, C., 'The interactions between inflammation and thrombosis', *British Journal of Haematology*, 131 (2005), pp. 417–30; Wise, J., 'Covid-19 and thrombosis: what do we know about the risks and treatment?', *British Medical Journal*, (2020), p. 369.

53 Meier, T. et al, 'Cardiovascular mortality attributable to dietary risk factors in 51 countries in the WHO European Region from 1990–2016: a systematic analysis of the Global Burden of Disease Study', *European Journal of Epidemiology*, 34 (2019), pp. 37–55.

54 Virani, S. et al, 'Heart disease and stroke statistics, 2020 Update: A report from the American Heart Association', *Circulation*, 141:9 (2020).

55 Shrivastava, A. et al, 'C-reactive protein, inflammation and coronary heart disease', *The Egyptian Heart Journal*, 67:2 (2015), pp. 89–97; Ridker, P. et al, 'Anti-inflammatory therapy with Canakinumab for atherosclerotic disease', *New England Journal of Medicine*, 377 (2017), pp. 1119–31.

56 Gutkowska, J. and Jankowski, M., 'Oxytocin: old hormone, new drug', *Pharmaceuticals*, 2 (2009), pp. 168–83.

57 Kiecolt-Glaser, J. et al, 'Close relationships, inflammation and health'.

58 Kuzawa, C. and Sweet, E., 'Epigenetics and the embodiment of race: developmental origins of US racial disparities in cardiovascular health', *American Journal of Human Biology*, 21 (2009), pp. 2–15; Pellanda, L. et al, 'Low birth weight and markers of inflammation and endothelial activation in adulthood', *International Journal of Cardiology*, 134:3 (2009), pp. 371–77.

59 Van de Maele, K. et al, 'In utero programming and early detection of cardiovascular disease in the offspring of mothers with obesity', *Atherosclerosis*, 275 (2018), pp. 182–95.

60 Meier, T. et al, 'Cardiovascular mortality attributable to dietary risk factors in 51 countries in the WHO European Region from 1990–2016'.

61 DiNicolantonio, J. and O'Keefe, J., 'Omega 6 vegetable oils as a driver of coronary heart disease: the oxidized linoleic acid hypothesis', *Open Heart*, 5:2 (2018), e000898.

62 Lustig, R., 'Sugar is the "alcohol of the child"', *Guardian* (4 January 2017).

63 Teodoro, J. et al, 'Therapeutic options targeting oxidative stress, mitochondrial dysfunction and inflammation to hinder the progression of vascular complications of diabetes', *Frontiers in Physiology*, 9 (2019), article 1857.

64 Inchauspe, J., *The Glucose Revolution* (Short Books, 2022).

65 Milei, J. et al, 'Perinatal and infant early atherosclerotic coronary lesions', *Canadian Journal of Cardiology*, 24:2 (2008); Guerri-Guttenberg, R. et al, 'Coronary intimal thickening begins in fetus and progresses in pediatric population and adolescents to atherosclerosis', *Angiology*, 71:1 (2019).

66 Linton, M. et al, 'The role of lipids and lipoproteins in atherosclerosis', in Feingold, K.R., Anawalt, B., Boyce, A. et al (eds.), Endotext [Internet]. South Dartmouth (MA): MDText.com, Inc.; 2000, 2019.

67 Epure, A. et al, 'Risk factors during first 1,000 days of life for carotid intima media thickness in infants, children and adolescents: a systematic review with meta-analyses', *PLOS Medicine*, 17:11 (2020), e1003414;

Rerkasem, K. et al, 'Intrauterine nutrition and carotid intima media thickness in young Thai adults', *Asia Pacific Journal of Clinical Nutrition*, 21:2 (2012), pp. 247–52; Gale, C. et al, 'Maternal diet during pregnancy and carotid intima-media thickness in children', *Arteriosclerosis, Thrombosis and Vascular Biology*, 26:8 (2006), pp. 1877–82.

68 Wunsch, R. et al, 'Intima media thickness in obese children before and after weight loss', *Pediatrics*, 118:6 (2006), article 23342340; Neuhauser, H. et al, 'Carotid intima media thickness percentiles in adolescence and young adulthood and their association with obesity and hypertensive blood pressure in a population cohort', *Hypertension*, 79:6 (2022), pp. 1167–76.

69 Van de Maele, K. et al, 'In utero programming and early detection of cardiovascular disease in the offspring of mothers with obesity'; Hakulinen, C. et al, 'Childhood psychosocial cumulative risks and carotid intima-media thickness in adulthood', *Psychosomatic Medicine*, 78:2 (2016), pp. 171–81; Juonala, M. et al, 'Influence of age on associations between childhood risk factors and carotid intima-media thickness in adulthood', *Circulation*, 122 (2010), pp. 2514–20.

70 Kothapalli, D. et al, 'Cardiovascular protection by ApoE and ApoE-HDL linked to suppression of ECM gene expression and arterial stiffening', *Cell Reports*, 2:5 (2012), pp. 1259–71.

71 Murphy, M. et al, 'Developmental origins of cardiovascular disease: impact of early life stress in humans and rodents', *Neuroscience and Biobehavioral Reviews*, 74:Pt B (2017), pp. 543–65.

72 Thurston, R. et al, 'Abuse and subclinical cardiovascular disease among midlife women', *Stroke*, 45:8 (2014), pp. 2246–51.

73 Scott, K. et al, 'Association of childhood adversities and early-onset mental disorders with adult onset chronic physical conditions', *Archives of General Psychiatry*, 68:8 (2011), pp. 838–44.

74 Hamer, M. et al, 'Cortisol responses to mental stress and the progression of coronary artery calcification in healthy men and women', *Plos ONE*, 7:2 (2012), e31356; Seldenrijk, A. et al, 'Psychological distress, cortisol stress response and subclinical coronary calcification', *Psychoneuroendocrinology*, 37:1 (2012), pp. 48–55.

75 Valenti, V. et al, 'A 15-year warranty period for asymptomatic individuals without coronary artery calcium: a prospective follow up of 9715 individuals', *JACC Cardiovascular Imaging*, 8:8 (2015), pp. 900–9.

76 Juonala, M. et al, 'Influence of age on associations between childhood risk factors and carotid intima-media thickness in adulthood', *Circulation*, 122 (2010), pp. 2514–20.

77 Keinan-Boker et al 2009, quoted in Miller et al (2011).

78 Kelly-Irving, M. et al, 'Childhood adversity as a risk for cancer: findings from the 1958 British birth cohort survey'.

79 Anderson, S. and Whitaker, R., 'Attachment security and obesity in pre-school-aged children', *Archives of Pediatric and Adolescent Medicine*, 165:3 (2011), pp. 235–42.

80 Reuter, S. et al, 'Oxidative stress, inflammation, and cancer: how are they linked?', *Free Radical Biology and Medicine*, 49:11 (2010), pp. 1603–16.

81 Lu, H. et al, 'Inflammation, a key event in cancer development', *Molecular Cancer Research*, 4:4 (2006); Hussain, S. and Harris, C., 'Inflammation and cancer: an ancient link with novel potentials', *International Journal of Cancer*, 121:11 (2007), pp. 2373–80.

82 Kiecolt-Glaser, J. et al, 'Close relationships, inflammation and health'; Grivennikov, S. and Karin, M., 'Inflammatory cytokines in cancer: TNF and IL-6 take the stage', *Annals of the Rheumatic Diseases*, 70 (2011), i104–i108.

83 Menard, C. et al, 'Immune and neuroendocrine mechanisms of stress vulnerability and resilience'.

84 Russek, L. and Schwartz, G., 'Feelings of parental caring predict health status midlife: a 35-year follow-up of the Harvard Mastery of Stress Study', *Journal of Behavioural Medicine*, 20:1 (1997), pp. 1–13.

85 Fairbank, E. et al, 'Social support and c-reactive protein in a Quebec population cohort of children and adolescents', *PLoS ONE*, 17:6 (2022), e0268210; Costanzo, E. et al, 'Psychosocial factors and interleukin-6 among women with advanced ovarian cancer', *Cancer*, 104:2 (2005), pp. 305–13.

86 Puig, J. et al, 'Predicting adult physical illness from infant attachment: a prospective longitudinal study', *Health Psychology*, 32:4 (2013), pp. 409–17.

87 Hambrick, E. et al, 'Beyond the ACE score: examining relationships between timing of developmental adversity, relational health and developmental outcomes in children'.

88 Li, T. et al, 'Approaches mediating oxytocin regulation of the immune system', *Frontiers in immunology*, 7 (2017), article 693.

89 Buemann, B. and Uvnas-Moberg, K., 'Oxytocin may have a therapeutical potential against cardiovascular disease', *Medical Hypotheses*, 138 (2020), article 109597.

90 Baker, M. et al, 'Early rearing history influences oxytocin receptor epigenetic regulation in rhesus macaques', *PNAS*, 114:44 (2017), pp. 11769–774; Ellis, B. et al, 'Developmental programming of oxytocin through variation in early-life stress: four meta-analyses and a theoretical re-interpretation', *Clinical Psychology Review*, 86 (2021), article 101985.

91 Toepfer, P. et al, 'A role of oxytocin receptor gene brain tissue expression quantitative trait locus rs237895 in the intergenerational transmission of the effects of maternal child maltreatment', *Journal of the American Academy of Child and Adolescent Psychiatry*, 58 (2019); Feldman, R. et al, 'Parental oxytocin and early caregiving jointly shape children's oxytocin response and social reciprocity', *Neuropsychopharmacology*, 38 (2013), pp. 1154–62; Strathearn, L., 'Maternal neglect: oxytocin, dopamine and the neurobiology of attachment', *Neuroendocrinology*, 23 (2011), pp. 1054–65; Eapen, V. et al, 'Separation anxiety, attachment and interpersonal representation: disentangling the role of oxytocin in the perinatal period', *PLoS ONE* (2014).

92 Baker, M. et al, 'Early rearing history influences oxytocin receptor epigenetic regulation in rhesus macaques'; Gouin, J. et al, 'Associations among oxytocin receptor gene DNA methylation in adulthood, exposure to early life adversity, and childhood trajectories of anxiousness', *Scientific Reports*, 7 (2017), p. 7446.

93 Joushi, S. et al, 'Environmental enrichment and intranasal oxytocin administration reverse maternal separation-induced impairments of prosocial choice behaviour', *Pharmacology Biochemistry and Behavior*, 213 (2022).

94 Guastella, A., 'The effect of oxytocin nasal spray on social interaction in children with autism: a randomized clinical trial', *Molecular Psychiatry*, 28 (2023), pp. 834–42; Yatawara, C. et al, 'The effect of oxytocin nasal spray on social interaction deficits observed in young children with autism: a randomized clinical crossover trial', *Molecular Psychiatry*, 21:9 (2016), pp. 1225–31.

95 Ellis, B. et al, 'Developmental programming of oxytocin through variation in early-life stress: four meta-analyses and a theoretical re-interpretation'.

96 Buemann, B. and Uvnas-Moberg, K., 'Oxytocin may have a therapeutical potential against cardiovascular disease'.

7. Child poverty and health

1 Bukhman, G. et al, 'The Lancet NCDI Poverty Commission: bridging a gap in universal health coverage for the poorest billion', *The Lancet Commissions*, 396:10256 (2020), pp. 991–1044.

2 McGarvey, D., *Poverty Safari: Understanding the Anger of Britain's Underclass* (Arcade Publishing, 2020).

3 Cooper, C., 'Why poverty is like a disease', *Nautilus* (17 April 2017).

4 Monroe, J., 'Poverty has left me unable to open my own front door', *Guardian* (10 December 2014).

5 Tirado, L., *Hand to Mouth: The Truth About Being Poor in a Wealthy World* (Virago Press, 2014).

6 Lewis, P. et al, 'Reading the Riots', *Guardian/LSE report*, 2011.

7 Bradford, B. and Shiner, M., *Viewed with Suspicion: The human cost of stop and search in England and Wales*, Open Society Justice Initiative and StopWatch, 2013.

8 quoted in Marmot, M., *The Health Gap: The Challenge of an Unequal World* (Bloomsbury, 2015).

9 Lockwood, K. et al, 'Early-life socioeconomic status associates with interleukin-6 responses to acute laboratory stress in adulthood', *Physiology and Behaviour*, 188 (2018), pp. 212–20.

10 Zilioli, S. et al, 'SES, perceived control, diurnal cortisol and physical symptoms', *Psychoneuroendocrinology*, 75 (2017), pp. 36–43.

11 Turiano, N. et al, 'Perceived control reduces mortality risk at low, not high, education levels', *Health Psychology*, 33:8 (2014), pp. 883–90.

12 Zilioli, S. et al, 'Life satisfaction moderates the impact of socioeconomic status on diurnal cortisol slope', *Psychoneuroendocrinology*, 60 (2015), pp. 91–5.

13 Williams, R., quote from *The World's Greatest Dad* (2009), screenplay by Bob Goldthwait.

14 Coussons-Read, M. et al, 'Psychosocial stress increases inflammatory markers and alters cytokine production across pregnancy', *Brain, Behaviour and Immunity*, 21 (2007), pp. 343–50; Uchino, B., 'Social support and health: a review of physiological processes potentially underlying links to disease outcomes', *Journal of Behavioral Medicine*, 29:4 (2006).

15 Uchino, B., 'Social support and health: a review of physiological processes potentially underlying links to disease outcomes'; Grewen, K., 'Effects of partner support on resting oxytocin, cortisol, norepinephrine and blood pressure before and after warm partner contact', *Psychosomatic Medicine*, 67:4 (2005), pp. 531–8.

16 Onaka, T. and Takayanagi, Y., 'Role of oxytocin in the control of stress and food intake', *Journal of Neuroendocrinology*, 31:3 (2019).

17 John-Henderson, N. et al, 'Socioeconomic status and social support: social support reduces inflammatory reactivity for individuals whose early-life socioeconomic status was low', *Psychological Science*, (2015), pp. 1–10.

18 Badrick, E. et al, 'The relationship between smoking status and cortisol secretion'.

19 McEvoy, C. and Spindel, E., 'Pulmonary effects of maternal smoking on the fetus and child: effects on lung development, respiratory morbidities, and life-long lung health', *Paediatric Respiratory Review*, 21 (2017), pp. 27–33.

20 Holz, N. et al, 'The long-term impact of early life poverty on orbitofrontal cortex volume in adulthood: results from a prospective study over 25 years', *Neuropsychopharmacology*, 40:4 (2015), pp. 996–1004.

21 Tryon, M. et al, 'Excessive sugar consumption may be a difficult habit to break: a view from the brain and body', *Journal of Clinical Endocrinology and Metabolism*, 100:6 (2015), pp. 2239–47.

22 Onaka, T. and Takayanagi, Y., 'Role of oxytocin in the control of stress and food intake'.

23 Piontak, J. et al, 'Violence exposure and adolescents' same-day obesogenic behaviours', *Social Science and Medicine*, 189 (2017), pp. 145–51.

24 Bentley, A. et al, 'Recent origin and evolution of obesity-income correlation across the United States', *Palgrave Communications*, 4 (2018), article 146; Foster, H. et al, 'Chapter 35 – Poverty/socioeconomic status and exposure to violence in the lives of children and adolescents', in *The Cambridge Handbook of Violent Behaviour and Aggression* (Cambridge University Press, 2012).

25 Volkow, N. et al, 'Imaging dopamine's role in drug abuse and addiction', *Neuropharmacology*, 56:1 (2009), pp. 3–8; Volkow, N. et al, 'Reward, dopamine and the control of food intake: implications for obesity', *Trends in Cognitive Sciences*, 15:1 (2011), pp. 37–46.

26 Evans, G., 'Childhood poverty and adult psychological well-being', *PNAS*, 113:52 (2016), pp. 14949–52.

27 Viner, R. et al, 'Responding to the changing burden of disease for children and adolescents in modern Britain: the RCPCH State of Child Health Report 2017', *BMJ Paediatrics Open*, 1:1 (2017), e000026.

28 Gillman, M. et al, 'Beverage intake during pregnancy and childhood adiposity', *Pediatrics*, 140:2 (2017), e20170031.

29 Mameli, C. et al, 'Nutrition in the first 1000 days: the origin of childhood obesity', *International Journal of Environmental Research and Public Health*, 13:838 (2016).

30 Bentley, A. et al, 'U.S. obesity as delayed effect of excess sugar', *Economics and Human Biology*, 36 (2020), article 100818.

31 Stanislawski, M. et al, 'Gut microbiota in the first 2 years of life and the association with BMI at age 12 in a Norwegian birth cohort', *American Society for Microbiology*, 9:5 (2018), e01751–18.

32 Hawkins, S. et al, 'Early in the life course: time for obesity prevention', in Halfon, N. et al (eds.), *Handbook of Life Course Health Development* (Springer, 2018).

33 Gibbs, B. and Forste, R., 'Socioeconomic status, infant feeding practices and early childhood obesity', *Paediatric Obesity*, 9:2 (2014), pp. 135–46; Huang, J. et al, 'Early feeding of larger volumes of formula milk is associated with greater body weight or overweight in later infancy', *Nutrition Journal*, 17:12 (2018); Michaelsen, K. and Greer, F., 'Protein needs early in life and long-term health', *American Journal of Clinical Nutrition*, 99:3 (2014) 718S–22S.

34 Ibid.

35 Grant, A. et al, '"People try and police your behaviour": the impact of surveillance on mothers' and grandmothers' perceptions and experiences of infant feeding', *Families Relationships and Societies*, 7:3 (2018), pp. 431–47.

36 Clarke, K. and Hier, S., 'Health and Wellbeing Breastfeeding Report Update, Brighton and Hove City Council' (2017); Blackpool Council, 'Healthy Beginnings for a Healthy Future', Appendix 4 d (2018); Peregrino, A. et al, 'Breastfeeding practices in the United Kingdom: is the neighbourhood context important?', *Maternal & Child Nutrition*, 14 (2018), e12626.

37 Thompson, A. and Bentley, M., 'The critical period of infant feeding for the development of early disparities in obesity', *Social Science and Medicine*, 97 (2013).

38 Ibid.

39 Nelson, M. et al, 'Low income diet and nutrition survey', commissioned by Food Standards Agency, The Stationery Office (2007); Cockroft, J. et al, 'Fruit and vegetable intakes in a sample of pre-school children participating in the "Five for All" project in Bradford', *Public Health and Nutrition*, 8:7 (2005), pp. 861–9.

40 NHS Health Survey for England, 2018.
41 Thompson, A. and Bentley, M., 'The critical period of infant feeding for the development of early disparities in obesity'.
42 Leermakers, E., 'Sugar containing beverage intake at the age of 1 year and cardiometabolic health at the age of 6 years', *International Journal of Behaviour, Nutrition and Physical Activity*, 12:114 (2015); Mameli, C. et al, 'Nutrition in the first 1000 days: the origin of childhood obesity', *International Journal of Environmental Research and Public Health*, 13 (2016), p. 838.
43 Baker, C., House of Commons Library Research Briefing, Obesity Statistics, 2023.
44 Bell, J. et al, 'Early metabolic features of genetic liability to type 2 diabetes: cohort study with repeated metabolomics across early life', *Diabetes Care*, 43:11 (2020).
45 Lambertz, J. et al, 'Fructose: a dietary sugar in crosstalk with microbiota contributing to the development and progression of non-alcoholic liver disease', *Frontiers in Immunology*, 8 (2017), p. 1159.
46 Wilson, B., 'Good enough to eat? The toxic truth about modern food', *Guardian* (16 March 2019).
47 Swinburn, B. et al, 'The global syndemic of obesity, undernutrition and climate change', *The Lancet Commissions*, 393:10173 (2019), pp. 791–846.
48 Trasande, L. et al, 'Food additives and child health', *Pediatrics*, 142:2 (2018).
49 Bentley, A. et al, 'U.S. obesity as delayed effect of excess sugar'.
50 Aeberli, I. et al, 'Fructose intake is a predictor of LDL particle size in overweight schoolchildren', *American Journal of Clinical Nutrition*, 86 (2007), pp. 1174–8.
51 Trafton, A., 'How mucus tames microbes', *Science Daily* (14 October 2019).
52 Lambertz, J. et al, 'Fructose: a dietary sugar in crosstalk with microbiota contributing to the development and progression of non-alcoholic liver disease'.

53 Evans, G., 'Stressing out the poor', *Pathways*, Winter 2011, Stanford Center on Poverty and Inequality, 2011.
54 Berlin, L., 'Correlates and consequences of spanking and verbal punishment for low-income White, African American and Mexican American toddlers', *Child Development*, 80:5 (2009), pp. 1403–20; Lee, Y., 'Adolescent motherhood and capital: interaction effects of race/ethnicity on harsh parenting', *Community Psychology*, 41:1 (2013, pp. 102–16; Hoff, E. et al, Bornstein, M. (ed.), 'SES and parenting', in *Handbook of Parenting*, vol. 2 (Erlbaum, 2002).
55 Tirado, L., *Hand to Mouth: The Truth About Being Poor in a Wealthy World*.
56 Van IJzendoorn, M. and Bakermans-Kranenburg, M., 'Invariance of adult attachment across gender, age, culture and socioeconomic status', *Journal of Social and Personal Relationships*, 27:2 (2010), pp. 200–8.
57 Kakinami, L. et al, 'Parenting style and obesity risk in children', *Preventive Medicine*, 75 (2015), pp. 18–22.
58 Anderson, S. and Whitaker, R., 'Attachment security and obesity in pre-school-aged children'.
59 Beeber, L. et al, 'Depressive symptoms and compromised parenting in low-income mothers of infants and toddlers: distal and proximal risks', *Research in Nursing and Health*, 37:4 (2014), pp. 276–91.
60 Clearfield, M. and Jedd, K., 'The effects of socio-economic status on infant attention', *Infant and Child Development*, 22:1 (2012), pp. 53–67.
61 Betancourt, L. et al, 'Effect of SES disparity on neural development in female African-American babies aged one month', *Developmental Science*, 19:6 (2016), pp. 947–56.
62 Hanson, J. et al, 'Family Poverty affects the rate of human infant brain growth', *PLoS ONE*, 8:12 (2013), e80954.
63 Holz, N. et al, 'The long-term impact of early life poverty on orbitofrontal cortex volume in adulthood: results from a prospective study over 25 years'.
64 Katz, I. et al, 'The relationship between parenting and poverty', York: The Joseph Rowntree Foundation, 2007; Evans, G., 'Stressing out the

poor', *Pathways*, Winter 2011, Stanford Center on Poverty and Inequality, 2011.

65 Johnson, M. et al, 'The relationship between maternal responsivity, SES, and resting autonomic nervous system functioning in Mexican American children', *International Journal of Psychophysiology* (2017).

66 Buckner, J. et al, 'Self-regulation and its relations to adaptive functioning in low income youths', *American Journal of Orthopsychiatry*, 79:1 (2009), pp. 19–30.

67 Luecken, L. et al, 'A longitudinal study of the effects of child-reported maternal warmth on cortisol stress response 15 years after divorce', *Psychosomatic Medicine*, 78:2 (2016), pp. 163–70.

68 Chen, E. et al, 'Maternal warmth buffers the effects of low early-life socio-economic status on pro-inflammatory signalling in adulthood', *Molecular Psychiatry*, 16:7 (2011), pp. 329–37.

69 Miller, G. et al, 'Psychological stress in childhood and susceptibility to the chronic diseases of aging: moving towards a model of behavioural and biological mechanisms'.

70 Berger, E. et al, 'Multi cohort study identifies social determinants of systemic inflammation over the life course', *Nature Communications*, 10:773 (2019).

71 Liu, R. et al, 'Socioeconomic status in childhood and C-reactive protein in adulthood: a systematic review and meta-analysis', *Journal of Epidemiology and Community Health*, 71:8 (2017), pp. 817–26.

72 Carroll, J. et al, 'Early childhood socioeconomic status is associated with circulating interleukin-6 among mid-life adults', *Brain, Behavior and Immunity*, 25 (2011), pp. 1468–74; Ziol-Guest, K. et al, 'Early childhood poverty, immune-mediated disease processes, and adult productivity', *PNAS*, 109 (2012), pp. 17289–93.

73 Kay, J., 'Our poor excuse for an understanding of poverty', *Financial Times*, 19 June 2012.

74 Chapman, J., 'Why higher benefits won't solve child poverty', *Mail Online* (31 January 2013).

75 Gillies, V. et al, 'Brave new brains: sociology, family and the politics of knowledge', *The Sociological Review*, 64 (2016), pp. 219–37.

76 Taylor, B. et al, 'Experiences of social work intervention among mothers with perinatal mental health needs', *Health and Social Care in the Community*, 27:6 (2019), pp. 1586–96.
77 Wahlbeck, K. et al, 'Interventions to mitigate the effects of poverty and inequality on mental health', *Social Psychiatry and Psychiatric Epidemiology*, 52:1 (2017).
78 Akee, R. et al, 'Parents' incomes and children's outcomes: a quasi-experiment using transfer payments from casino profits', *American Economic Journal: Applied Economics*, 2 (2010); Yoshikawa, H. et al, 'The effects of poverty on the mental, emotional and behavioural health of children and youth', *American Psychologist* (May–June 2012).
79 Duncan, G., 'Income supplements for parents of young children could tackle entrenched long-term inequalities', Child and Family Blog, 2014.

Conclusion

8. Future-proofing human beings

1 Nash, M. et al, 'Early microbes modify immune system development and metabolic homeostasis – the "restaurant" hypothesis revisited', *Frontiers in Endocrinology* (13 December 2017).
2 Martin, S. et al, 'Is an ounce of prevention worth a pound of cure? A cross-sectional study of the impact of English public health grant on mortality and morbidity', *BMJ Open*, 10 (2020), e036411.
3 'GMC is criticised for investments in Nestlé and McDonald's', *British Medical Journal*, 380 (2023), p. 580.
4 Ungoed-Thomas, J. et al, ' "It's naïve to think this is in the best interests of the NHS." How Big Pharma's millions are influencing health care', *Observer* (8 July 2023).
5 Knox 2014, 'The blame and shame society', *Psychoanalytic Psychotherapy* 28 (3): 244–8, 2014.
6 Perks, B., Blogsite: 'Because I grew up in an orphanage', 2019
7 Crump,C. and Howell,E., 'Perinatal origins of cardiovascular health disparities across the life course', *JAMA Pediatrics* 174 (2):113–14, 2020;

Schaaf, J. et al, 'Ethnic and racial disparities in the risk of preterm birth: a systematic review and meta-analysis', *American Journal of Perinatologyy* 30 (06):433–50, 2013.

8   Iacobucci, G., 'Medical model of care needs updating, say experts', *British Medical Journal*, 360 (2018).

9   Gilbert, S. and Green, C., *Vaxxers: A Pioneering Moment in Scientific History* (Hodder & Stoughton, 2021).

10 Simon, M., *Appetite for Profit: How the Food Industry Undermines Our Health and How to Fight Back* (Nation Books, 2006).

11 Costanza, R. et al, 'Overcoming societal addictions: what can we learn from individual therapies?', *Ecological Economics*, 131 (2017), pp. 543–50.

12 Halfon, N. et al, 'Lifecourse health development: past, present and future', *Maternity and Child Health Journal*, 18 (2014), pp. 344–65.

13 Public Health England, 'Health matters: health and work', 2019.

14 Integrated Benefits Institute, 2017.

15 Full Fact, 'How much of the NHS budget is spent on treating chronic conditions?' (25 May 2011).

16 Renfrew, M. et al, 'Preventing disease and saving resources: the potential contribution of increasing breastfeeding rates in the UK', UNICEF UK, 2012.

17 Vareki, S. et al, 'Moving on from Metchnikoff: thinking about microbiome therapeutics in cancer', *ecancermedicalscience* 12 (2018), p. 867.

18 Kendrick, M., *The Clot Thickens: The Enduring Mystery of Heart Disease* (Columbus Publishing, 2021).

19 Angelis, A. et al, 'Promoting population health through pharmaceutical policy', LSE, 2023.

20 Brittain, H. et al, 'The rise of the genome and personalised medicine', *Clinical Medicine* (London) 17:6 (2017), pp. 545–51.

21 HM Government, 'Genome UK: the future of healthcare', 2020.

22 Hanson, M. and Gluckman, P., 'Developmental origins of noncommunicable disease: population and public health implications', *American Journal of Clinical Nutrition*, 94:6 (2011), 1754S–1758S.

Notes

23 Gottlieb, G., 'Probabilistic epigenesis', *Developmental Science*, 10:1 (2007), pp. 1–11; Cohen, I. and Harel, D., 'Explaining a complex living system: dynamics, multi-scaling and emergence', *Journal of the Royal Society Interface*, 4:13 (2007), pp. 175–82.

24 Huber, M. et al, 'How should we define health?' *British Medical Journal*, 343 (2011), d4163.

25 Royal College of Midwives (RCM) press release, 'Maternity underfunding means care is based on what trusts can afford not on women's safety and needs', March 2022.

26 Institute of Health Visiting press release, 'Public health grant settlement – not enough to deliver the "best start in life"', February 2024.

27 Rimmer, A., 'Child health: government must act now to increase investment in services, says BMA', *British Medical Journal*, 368, 2020.

28 Persson, P. and Rossin-Slater, M., 'When Dad can stay home: fathers' workplace flexibility and maternal health', National Bureau of Economic Research working paper 25902 (2019).

29 Plotka, R. and Busch-Rossnagal, N., 'The role of length of maternity leave in supporting mother-child interactions and attachment security among American mothers and their infants', *International Journal of Child Care and Education Policy*, 12 (2018), article 2.

30 Hashemi, L. et al, 'Exploring the health burden of cumulative and specific adverse childhood experiences in New Zealand: results from a population-based study'.

31 Thackeray, W. M., *Vanity Fair* (Bradbury & Evans, 1848).

Epigraph and image credits

Epigraphs

The epigraphs in this book have been reproduced from the following sources, with thanks to the authors:

P. 11: *The Master and His Emissary: The Divided Brain and the Making of the Western World*, copyright © 2009 Iain McGilchrist, reproduced with permission of the Licensor through PLSclear; p. 33: 'President Obama & Marilynne Robinson: A Conversation in Iowa', *New York Review of Books*, Nov 15 2015. Copyright © 2015 President Barack Obama and Marilynne Robinson; p. 61: Cohen Irun R and Harel David. 'Explaining a complex living system: dynamics, multi-scaling and emergence'. *J. R. Soc. Interface*. 4: 175–182 (2007), //doi.org/10.1098/rsif.2006.0173; p. 73: *Ariel: Poems* by Sylvia Plath, Faber and Faber Ltd (1965); p. 139: *Collected Poems* by Philip Larkin, Faber and Faber Ltd (2003); p. 139: 'The Pact' from *The Dead and The Living* by Sharon Olds, copyright © 1975, 1978, 1979, 1980, 1981, 1982, 1983 by Sharon Olds. Used by permission of Alfred A. Knopf, an imprint of the Knopf Doubleday Publishing Group, a division of Penguin Random House LLC. All rights reserved; p. 167: *Poverty Safari: Understanding the Anger of Britain's Underclass*, first published in 2018 by Picador, in association with Luath Press Limited. Picador is an imprint of Pan Macmillan. Reproduced by permission of Macmillan Publishers International Limited. Copyright © Darren McGarvey 2017; p. 167: *The Health Gap: The Challenge of an Unequal World*, copyright © Michael Marmot 2015, Bloomsbury Publishing Plc; p. 195: *The Rise And Fall Of Modern Medicine*, copyright © 1999, 2011, by James Le Fanu, reproduced with permission of the Licensor through PLSclear.

Epigraph and image credits

Images

P. 19: © American Philosophical Society; p. 40: reproduced by kind permission of Professor Alan Sroufe; p. 45: reproduced by kind permission of Dr Allan Schore; p. 47: New America, 2014, reproduced under Creative Commons License 2.0; p. 56: reproduced by kind permission of the family of Professor David Barker; p. 62: Free Range Projects at 777 International Mall, Miami, 2018 © Tschabalala Self; p. 64: Bill Coster IN / Alamy Stock Photo, Image ID: AHYYW6 (RM); p. 79: image reproduced by kind permission of Dr Elseline Hoekzema; p. 82: © South Schleswig Voter Federation; p. 86: Nicolas Guyonnet / AFP via Getty Images, Image ID: 2156713394; p. 93: Too young to drink, 2017 © European Fetal Alcohol Spectrum Disorders Alliance; p. 102: taken from 'Mother Protects Duckling from Hungry Crow' © Bruce Causer, www.youtube.com/watch?v=xmaY2opcTuY; p. 104: from the author's collection; p. 118: from the author's collection; p. 125: © Haberturk Journalism Inc; p. 127: from the author's collection; p. 142: reproduced by permission of Dr Vincent Felitti; p. 148: reproduced by kind permission of Professors Gregory Miller and Edith Chen; p. 150: © American Association for the Advancement of Science, 2014; p. 169: © Linda Tirado via X; p. 173: © North Tees and Hartlepool NHS Foundation Trust, 2017; p. 177: Compassionate Eye Foundation / David Oxberry / Photodisc via Getty Images, Image ID: 1045551084; p. 179: from 'Choosing sugary drinks over fruit juice for toddlers linked to risk of adult obesity', Ffion White, 2024; p. 182: © Zion Market Research, 2020; p. 211: Sure Start © *Surrey Advertiser*.

The author and publisher gratefully acknowledge the permission granted to reproduce the copyright material in this book. Every effort has been made to trace copyright holders and to obtain their permission. The publisher apologises for any errors or omissions and, if notified of any corrections, will make suitable acknowledgment in future reprints or editions of this book.

Acknowledgements

This has been a long project that has lasted several years. At its inception, Tom Thorpe, Vicki Cairns, Gillie Ruscombe-King and Mike Murphy encouraged me to think there was a book waiting to emerge. From the start, Jane Henriques was cheerleader-in-chief, consistently urging me to keep going despite obstacles.

As the work started to take shape, friends and colleagues Fiona Crosse, Sarah Stewart-Brown, Jane Barlow, Arthur King, Andrew Lea and Vivette Glover gave valuable detailed feedback on particular chapters. Thanks for their expertise. Thank you also to the numerous other amazing scientists whose years of research originated the work on which the book draws. In the later phases of the project, special thanks go to those who were kind enough to find the time to read and comment on the whole manuscript: Joanna Tucker, Mike Murphy, Jean Knox, Doro Marden, Melanie Chait and Rita Carter.

Various people in the publishing world were also midwives to the book. Via The Writing Coach, run by Jacqui Lofthouse and Jacqueline Smith, Susan Watt helped me see the manuscript through a fresh pair of eyes. My agent, Sam Copeland at Rogers Coleridge and White, supported and launched the book, finding a good home for it with Cornerstone (Penguin Random House), where the book was championed by my editor, Anna Argenio. Her astute insights and suggestions sometimes surprised me but made a difference. She was assisted by Matilda Oduntan, who offered further useful fine-tuning and help with many of the practicalities involved in bringing the project to completion. Others at Penguin Random House also contributed, including Helen Conford, publisher at Cornerstone Press and Rose Waddilove, the managing editor, who held

Acknowledgements

the fort until Elena Roberts came on board to provide further editorial guidance and reassurance. Anna Herve did a great job of copy-editing, making further valuable improvements. Finally, Ania Gordon, the marketing manager, publicity director Rachel Kennedy and cover designer Lucy Thorne were an essential part of the process. In Oxford, Steve Preston gave me much-needed technological support.

I am also grateful to all those who offered emotional support and re-fuelling, sustaining me over a period of years as I researched and wrote at an ever slower pace: Gillian Swanson, Chris Shingler, Joanna Dennison, Jane Henriques, Sue Weaver, Barbara Burke, Wendy Davies, Sally Baden, Fiona Crosse, Gillie Ruscombe-King, Jean Knox, Lorna Smalley and Roger Smalley, Doro Marden and Leslie Sklair, Melanie Chait, David Glyn, Graham Music, Caroline Merry, Sohani Hayhurst, Mollie Kenyon-Jones, Ian Maskell, Michele Topham, Richard Parsons, Helen King and Margaret Landale.

Above all, thanks to my kind and steadfast family: Jess Aspinall and Nick Murteira, Laurie Gerhardt and Chiara Jancke, and Vicky Aspinall.

Index

Action on Smoking and Health (ASH), 95
ADHD, 87, 95
adrenaline, 47
adverse childhood experiences (ACEs), 3, 44, 49–52, 139–50, 211–12
   depression and, 144–5, 147
   gut microbiome and, 154
   humiliation, 3, 143, 146
   inflammation and, 147, 154, 163
   life expectancy and, 143
   neglect, 50, 124, 143
   obesity and, 141–4, 174, 184–7
   oxytocin and, 124, 164–6
   parenting and, 212
   physical abuse, 46, 143, 144, 146
   physical health and, 143–50, 160–61, 163, 180
   regulation and, 46, 131, 134–5, 140
   serotonin and, 128
   sexual abuse, 140–44
   stress response and, 44, 49–52, 131, 135
affective neuroscience, 65
ageing, 6, 69, 160
   ACEs and, 145, 160
   chronic conditions and, 204, 209
   epigenetic alterations and, 26
   longevity, 143, 171, 204–5
Ainsworth, Mary, 37
alcohol, 19, 82, 90–94, 128, 144
allergies, 109–10, 150
Alzheimer's disease, 30, 153
amygdala, 45, 77, 98, 124, 127, 135
Anda, Robert, 141, 143–4, 166

antibiotics, 16–17, 109
antioxidants, 151
anxiety, 49, 51
   ACEs and, 145, 147
   core routines, 65
   fetal development and, 92, 98
   microbiome and, 107
   omega-3 and, 126
   oxytocin and, 105, 123–4, 126, 165
   serotonin and, 127
Arnott, Deborah, 95
arthritis, 27
asthma, 95
Astra-Zeneca, 201
atherosclerosis, 154, 156, 159, 183
attachment relationships, *see under* relationships
attachment theory, 37
Attenborough, David, 200
authoritarian parenting, 36, 46, 184–7
autism, 123
auto-immune conditions, 109, 150
autonomic nervous system, 77

'baby boomer' generation, 2
Baby Clubs, 121
bacteria, 16–17, 63, 75, 80, 105
   microbiome, 5, 42, 52, 78, 90, 106–13, 175
Bakan, Joel, 202
Bandoli, Gretchen, 93
Barboza Solis, Cristina, 145
Barker, David, 55–56, 84, 159
Bengtsson, Jessica, 146

Index

Bentley, Margaret, 179
Berkeley Guidance Study, 36
Best Beginnings, 210
Better Start, A, 210
Beveridge, William, 20
Biden, Joe, 190
bifidobacteria, 78, 107–8, 113
Big Pharma, 196, 201
birth cohort studies, 36, 38, 54, 84
birth rates, 54, 204–5
Biswas, Subrata, 151
blood pressure, 3, 17, 53, 80, 84–5, 125–6
Body Mass Index (BMI), 80, 85, 88, 175, 188
body weight, 3, 4, 30, 43, 51, 53, 80, 85–9, 99, 151, 173–87
   ACEs and, 141–3, 144, 174, 184–7
   breastfeeding and, 176–8
   fetal development and, 80, 85–9, 97, 99
   health risks, 180–81
   inflammation and, 85, 87, 152–5
   politics and, 181–3
   poverty and, 173–83, 199
Bowlby, John, 37
brain, 15, 105
   fetal development, 77–8, 98
   fight or flight response, 47–8, 103
   neural connections, 3, 39, 45, 78, 79
   neuron cells, 69
   neurotransmitters, 5, 65, 105, 132–3
   oxytocin and, 124
   SEEKING system, 65
brain reserve, 3
breastfeeding, 4, 78, 103, 105–9, 112, 114–23, 151, 176–8, 205
   immune system and, 114–17, 151, 198–9
   microbiome and, 106–9, 175
   obstacles to, 117–19
   omega-3 fatty acids, 125–6
   politics of, 119–23

   poverty and, 176–8, 184
   stress and, 25–6, 50, 107
breasts, 119–20
Bronfenbrenner, Urie, 37
Brown, Julia and Simon, 92
Bruer, John, 42–3
Buck, Carrie, 20
Buemann, Ben, 165–6
Burr, Vivien, 70–71
butyrate, 109–11, 154

cancers, 1–2, 17, 98, 99, 161–2
   ACEs and, 144, 154, 161
   breastfeeding and, 117, 120
   chemotherapy, 12, 17, 206
   epigenetic alterations and, 26
   inflammation and, 154–5, 162
   microbiome and, 154, 205–6
Cannon, Ellie, 122
capitalism, 30, 70–71, 202
cardiovascular disease, 2–4, 17, 51, 98–9, 156–61, 180
   ACEs and, 143–4, 147, 154, 160
   fetal nutrition and, 57, 81–2, 84
   microbiome and, 15–5
Carolinska Institute, 88
Caspi, Avshalom, 53
cells, 61–71
   fat cells, 88–9
   fetal development, 66–7, 71, 74
   immune system, 114
   stem cells, 67–71
Centre for Parenting Culture Studies, 42
Chadwick, Edwin, 34
Chain, Ernst, 16
Chatzi, Vaia, 88
Chen, Edith, 148
chick embryo experiment, 40–41
chickenpox, 115
child guidance movement (1920s–30s), 36–7

Index

Child Poverty Action Group, 189
Child Trauma Academy, 146
cholesterol, 53, 76, 78, 158, 160, 180, 183
chronic conditions, 2, 30, 32, 99, 196, 203
    ACEs and, 143–4
    ageing population and, 204, 209
    oxidants and, 151
    stress and, 51–4
chronic fatigue, 146–7
chronic obstructive pulmonary disease (COPD), 2, 143–4, 208, 214
Clearfield, Melissa, 186
climate overheating, 6, 209, 215
coeliac disease, 109
Cohen, I., 61
Cohen, Sheldon, 148–9
colic, 113
community health centres, 213
competition, 70–71
congenital heart disease (CHD), 83
Cooley, Charles, 34
Copenhagen, Denmark, 117–18
core routines, 65
coronary artery calcification (CAC), 160–61
Corporation, The (Bakan), 202
cortisol, 46–9, 51, 89, 94–5, 98, 148, 160, 171–2
Covid-19, 15, 155–6
Cow and Gate, 121
cowpox, 15
Cribsheet (Oster), 122
Crick, Francis, 21
crows, 102–3
CRP, 52, 54, 171, 188
Cryan, John, 109
cystic fibrosis, 22
cytokines, 52, 107, 110, 114, 149–52, 155, 162, 172

Damasio, Antonio, 70, 109
Danese, Andrea, 53–4
Darwin, Charles, 35, 55, 64
Decade of the Child (1920s), 35, 57
DeJong, Erica, 155
dementia, 3, 30, 149–50, 155
dendritic cells, 114
Dennett, Daniel, 71
depression, 3, 4, 27, 98
    ACEs and, 144–7
    inflammation and, 154
    microbiome and, 107
    poverty and, 170, 185, 199
    serotonin and, 128–9
Developing Genome, The (Moore), 25
developmental approach, 4–5, 31, 34, 37–40, 44, 57–8, 198
    attachment theory, 37
    birth cohort studies, 36, 38, 54
    developmental origins of health and disease (DoHD) hypothesis, 54–6
    stress and, 46–54
    timing, 40–43, 146
diabetes
    gestational, 85
    type 1, 109, 116, 146
    type 2, *see* type 2 diabetes
diet; nutrition, 3–4, 13, 144, 173–87, 196, 199, 202, 208
    infancy, 105–26, 178–9, 205
    inflammation and, 154–8, 180–81, 183
    politics and, 181–3
    poverty and, 173–83
    pregnancy, 54–5, 74, 76, 81–9, 96
    stress and, 141–3, 172, 173–87
Dinan, Ted, 109, 111
diseases of affluence, 17
DNA, 21–5, 68
    methylation, 24–5, 95
dopamine, 79, 126, 132, 174
Douglas, James, 54–5
drugs, medicines, 17–18, 29–30, 196–7, 201

Index

drugs, recreational, 53, 74, 82, 90–99, 172
Dubos, René, 5
ducks, 102–3
Duncan Smith, Iain, 188
Duncan, Greg, 190
Dunedin study, 38, 52–4
Dunn, Erin, 145
Dutch Hunger Winter (1944–5), 81–2
Dyke, Alex, 119

Ebola, 15
ecological systems theory, 38
egg cells, 57, 63, 66
Ein-Dor, Tsachi, 125
electroencephalogram (EEG), 29
emotions, regulation of, 45–6, 53, 65, 98, 127–9, 134–5, 140
   authoritarian parenting and, 186–7
   poverty and, 186–7
   smoking and, 173
endocrine system, 70, 105, 125, 182
Engels, Friedrich, 34
Enlightenment (c. 1685–1815), 30, 43
Entringer, Sonja, 89
environment, natural, 200
epigenetics, 24–7, 39, 57
   smoking and, 95
   stress and, 49, 57, 112
Essex, Marilyn, 49
eugenics, 18–21
evolution, 63–6, 69
exclusion, 96, 168
exercise, 6, 151, 157, 203

Fabian Society, 20
Family Nurse Partnership, 213
Felitti, Vincent, 90, 141–3, 142, 144, 147, 166
fetal alcohol syndrome (FAS), 92–4
fetal development, *see* pregnancy
fibromyalgia, 146

fight or flight response, 47–8, 103
Fleming, Alexander, 16
Florey, Howard, 16
food, *see* diet
food allergies, 109–10
formula milk, 106, 107–8, 113, 122, 176, 199, 201
four humours, 14
Fourth Industrial Revolution, 28
Franklin, Rosalind, 21
free radicals, 150–51
Freeman, George, 28–9
Freud, Anna, 35
Freud, Sigmund, 35, 142
Furman, Senta, 51

GABA, 132
Gagniere, Johan, 154
Garnham, Alison, 189
Gates, Bill, 203
Gay, Roxane, 144
General Medical Council, 197
genes, 18–27, 207
   determinism, 2–3
   DNA, 21–4
   epigenetics, 24–7, 39, 49
   eugenics, 18–21
genome-wide association studies (GWAS), 22
genomics, 29–30, 206
germ theory, 16–17
German measles, 115
Ghent University, 25
Glover, Vivette, 93
Gluckman, Peter, 94
glucocorticoid receptor genes, 25
Google, 28
Gordon, David, 170
Gottlieb, Gilbert, 207
green spaces, 151, 170
Gunnar, Megan, 46–7, 47
gut microbiome, *see* microbiome

270

Halfon, Neal, 203
Hall, Stanley, 35
Hambrick, Erin, 145–6
Hanson, Mark, 94
Harel, David, 61
Hartigan-O'Connor, Dennis, 115
Harvey, William, 14
Hawkins, Summer, 176
Head Start, 37, 43
health capital, 4, 198, 209
Health Gap, The (Marmot), 167, 168
health visitors, 35, 99, 108, 198, 210
healthcare, *see under* medicine
Healthy Child Programme, 210
heart, 76–7, 82–4, 95
   cardiovascular disease, *see* cardiovascular disease
   congenital conditions, 82–3
heroic thinking, 27
high-fructose corn syrup, 181, 201
high-tech approach, 28–31
Hippocrates, 14
Hoekzema, Elseline, 79, 79
Holmes, Oliver Wendell, 21
Holocaust (1941–5), 161
Holz, Natalie, 186–7
homeostasis, 43, 105
homophobia, 199
Hoover, Herbert, 36
hormones, 5–6, 105
   cortisol, 46–9, 51, 89, 94–5, 98, 148, 160, 171–3
   oestrogen, 74, 79
   oxytocin, 44, 123–7, 135
   serotonin, 95, 126–9, 132
Horton, Richard, 6
HPA axis, 48–9, 52, 111, 135, 147, 163, 172, 174
Human Genome Project, 22, 24–5
humiliation, 3, 143, 146
humoral theory, 14
Hunger (Gay), 144

Huntington's disease, 22
Huxley, Julian, 20

immune system, 2–3, 27, 42, 52, 53–4, 70, 105, 196
   ACEs and, 147–50, 163–4
   breastfeeding and, 114–17, 151, 198–9
   cholesterol and, 158
   fetal development of, 78–9
   microbiome and, 109–14
   stress and, 52–53, 111–12, 147–50
individualism, 23–4, 33, 96, 170, 181, 202
Industrial Revolution
   First (c. 1760–1840), 29, 34, 63–4
   Fourth (c. 2016–present), 28–9
inequality, 6, 96, 168, 208
infancy, 1, 6, 31, 34–43, 101–35
   ACEs, *see* adverse childhood experiences
   breastfeeding, *see* breastfeeding
   cohort studies, 36, 38, 54, 84
   microbiome during, 106–13, 175
   nutrition during, 105–26, 178–9, 205
   parenting, *see* parenting
   poverty and, 3, 34–5, 167–91
   regulation, emotional, 45–6, 53, 98, 127–9, 135, 140
   regulation, physiological, 43–6, 49–51, 129–33
   sensitive periods, 41–3, 146
   stress during, 26, 44, 46–54, 111, 139–50
inflammation, 3–4, 44, 52–4, 97, 148–56, 199, 215
   ACEs and, 147, 151, 163–4
   ageing and, 160
   cancers and, 154–155, 162
   coronavirus and, 155–6
   depression and, 154
   diet and, 154–5, 157–8, 180–81, 183
   fetal development and, 157
   microbiome and, 107, 109–13
   obesity and, 85, 87, 152–3, 155

inflammation – *cont.*
  omega-3 fatty acid and, 126, 150, 152–3
  oxytocin and, 165–6
  poverty and, 171–2, 188, 199
  sedentary lifestyles and, 157
  stress and, 52–4, 151, 154, 157, 171, 187
  vagal system and, 132
inflammatory bowel conditions, 154
informatics, 29
innate lymphoid cells (ILCs), 114
insulin, 83, 180–81
irritable bowel syndrome (IBS), 110
isolation, 171
Israel, 161

Jedd, Kelly, 186
Jemison, Ebony, 96
Jenner, Edward, 15, 16
Johnson, Sara, 105
Jones, Marshae, 96–7

Kaiser Permanente, 141–3
Kalisch-Smith, Jacinta, 83
Kanherkar, Riya, 50
Kellaway, Kate, 141
Kelly-Irving, Michelle, 162
Kendrick, Malcolm, 206
Keynes, John Maynard, 20
kidneys, 83, 98, 154
Kiecolt-Glaser, Janice, 149–50
King, Truby, 36
Klein, Melanie, 35
Knox, Jean, 134, 197
Komaroff, Anthony, 69

lactobacillus, 90, 107, 113
Lam, Birte Harlev, 210
Lancet, The, 6, 116, 181
Larkin, Philip, 139
Le Fanu, James, 195, 199
leukaemia 116
life expectancy, *see* longevity

Liu, Richard, 188
London riots (2011), 169
longevity, 143, 171, 204–5
López-Vicario, Cristina, 153
low-tech approach, 31–2
lungs, 53, 77–8, 89, 95, 98, 144, 155, 173
lymphoid structures, 110

malaria, 15
Marmot, Michael, 167, 168
Marshall, Martin, 197
Marshall, Nicole, 98
mast cells, 114
Master and His Emissary, The (McGilchrist), 11
mastitis, 117
Maté, Gabor, 123
maternity services, 99, 210
McGarvey, Darren, 167
McGilchrist, Iain, 11
measles, 15, 115
medication, 17–18
medicine, 13–18, 205–15
  care, 27
  drug culture, 17–18, 196–7, 201
  genetics and, 18–27
  high-tech approach, 28–31
  low-tech approach, 31–2
  personalised medicine, 29–30, 206
  prevention, 4, 13, 196–7, 207–15
  relationship-based care, 117
  'repair shop' model, 13, 205–6
Medicines and Healthcare products Regulatory Agency (MHRA), 197
Mendel, Gregor; Mendelian, 18, 35
mental health, 13, 51, 89–99
  ACEs and, 3–4, 51, 107, 144–5, 147
  inflammation and, 154
  microbiome and, 107
  parenting and, 143

Index

poverty and, 170, 185
pregnancy and, 89–99
serotonin and, 128–9
metabolic disorders, 84
methylation, 24–5, 95
microbiome, 5, 42, 52, 78, 90, 106–13, 164, 181, 196
    ACEs and, 154, 164
    cancers and, 154, 205–6
    immune system and, 109–14, 154
    inflammation and, 154–5, 181
    vagal system and, 132–3
microscopes, 15
midwives, 99, 117, 121, 210
milk
    breast milk, 105–9, 113–14, 121–2, 125
    formula milk, 106, 107–8, 113, 122, 125, 176, 199, 201
Miller, Gregory, 147–8, 149
Minnesota study, 38–9
Moffitt, Terrie, 53–4
Monroe, Jack, 168
Moore, David, 25, 27
Mortimer, Paul, 169
mucus gut lining, 110–11, 113–14, 154–5, 182
mumps, 115
myelin, 78
myeloma, 2

National Childbirth Trust, 122
National Health Service (NHS), 28, 31, 99, 173, 178, 196–7, 204, 210
natural killer (NK) cells, 114
nature versus nurture, 23–4, 27
Nazi Germany (1933–45), 21, 161
necrotising enterocolitis, 116
neonatal sepsis, 116
nephrons, 83
nerve cells, 15

nervous system, 47–8, 70, 77, 95
neural connections, 3, 39, 45, 78
neuro-inflammatory conditions, 126, 196, 208
neurological disease, 51
neurotransmitters, 5, 65, 105, 132, 133
neutrophils, 114
NICE, 197
nitric oxide, 157
non-communicable diseases (NCDs), 18, 98, 143–4, 207, 214
noradrenaline, 47
nutrition, *see* diet

Oakley, Laura, 119
Oaks, Brietta, 78n
obesity, *see* body weight
oestrogen, 74, 79
Olds, Sharon, 139–41
omega-3 fatty acids, 86–7, 106, 125, 150, 152–3
omega-6 fatty acids, 158
opioids, 17, 201
Orphan Drug Act (1983), 206
osteoporosis, 84
Oster, Emily, 122
oxidants, 150–52, 160, 180
OXPIP, 210
Oxycontin, 201
oxytocin, 44, 123–7, 135, 160, 164–6

Page, Lesley, 117
pancreas, 98
Panksepp, Jaak, 64–5
parenting, 3, 36–8, 45–6, 54, 101–4, 113, 199–200, 210–12
    abusive/neglectful, *see* adverse childhood experiences (ACEs)
    authoritarian, 36, 46, 184–7, 212
    egalitarian model, 101, 120, 211
    parental leave, 210–12
    poverty and, 184–7, 199, 212

parenting – *cont.*
  training model, 36, 46, 212
  warm/protective, 25, 104, 123–35, 162–6, 187–8, 198–200
Parkinson's disease, 2, 6, 113, 126, 153, 209
Pasteur, Louis, 16
Paynter, Nina, 23
peppered moths, 63–4
Perks, Benjamin, 197
Peyer's patches, 110
physical closeness, 25, 123–35
physiological regulation, 43–54
phytochemicals, 26
placenta, 74–6, 78–81
plants, 39, 61–2
plasticity, 40, 41
Plath, Sylvia, 73
Plomin, Robert, 23–4
polio, 15
politics, 200–203
  breastfeeding and, 119–23
  obesity and, 181–3
  poverty and, 188–91
pollution, 18, 57, 87–8, 96, 151, 157, 170, 199–201, 215
Porges, Steven, 44, 51, 129, 130, 135
poverty 3, 34–5, 95, 167–91, 199, 200, 206, 208
  health habits and, 172–83, 199
  mental health and, 170, 185, 199
  parenting and, 184–7, 199, 212
  politics and, 188–91
Poverty Safari (McGarvey), 168
power, 197
pre-eclampsia, 85
pregnancy; fetal development, 2, 4–5, 17, 28, 31, 41, 66–7, 71, 73–99, 210
  alcohol consumption during, 92–4
  body weight and, 80, 85–9, 97
  brain development, 77–8
  depression and, 98
  drug use during, 74–5, 82, 90–99

  hormones during, 74, 79
  immune system development, 78–9
  inflammation and, 157, 171
  microbiome development, 78, 90, 175
  neural networks and, 79
  nutrition during, 54–5, 57, 74, 76, 81–9, 96
  organ development, 76–7, 81–4, 95
  placenta, 74–6, 78–81
  pollution during, 87–8, 96
  smoking during, 172–3
  social networks and, 171
  stress during, 48–9, 57, 74, 75, 89–99, 157
prevention, 4, 13–15, 17–18, 30–32, 56, 58, 196–7, 207–9
progesterone, 74
protein, 83
psoriasis, 154
PTSD, 145
Public Health Grant, 210
Puig, Jennifer, 164

racism, 96, 168, 199, 206
Rea, Maeve, 155
regulation, 44–54, 125–35
  ACEs and, 146
  emotional, *see* emotions, regulation of
  oxytocin and, 125–6, 135
  serotonin and, 127–9, 132
  social self and, 133–5
  stress and, 46–54, 146
  vagal system and, 129–33
regulatory T-cells, 109
relationship-based care, 117
relationships, 37–8, 44, 49–51, 54, 105, 111–12, 137–50
  abusive/neglectful, *see* adverse childhood experiences
  immune system and, 111–12, 148–50, 157, 171–2

Index

nitric oxide and, 157
physical closeness, 25, 123–35
regulation and, 44–6, 49–51, 54, 123–35
social self and, 133–5, 171
vagal system and, 129–33
warm/protective, 25, 104, 123–35, 162–6, 172, 187–8, 198, 199–200
Repetti, Rena, 147
reproduction, 63
resolvins, 153
respiratory diseases, 143
responsibility, 96
rheumatoid arthritis, 109, 116, 154
rhinovirus, 149
Ribena, 113
riots, 169
Robinson, Marilynne, 33
Rockefeller family, 35
Royal College of Midwives, 210
Royal College of Paediatrics, 175
rubella, 82
Russell, Bertrand, 20

scarlet fever, 115
Schore, Allan, 44–5
Schulkin, Jay, 50
Scotland, 144
sedentary lifestyles, 18, 157
SEEKING system, 65
self-control, *see* emotions, regulation of
Sendak, Maurice, 105
sensitive periods, 41–3, 146
separation from parents, 3, 49, 65, 128
serotonin, 95, 126, 127–9, 132, 174
sexual abuse, 140–44
Shields, Brooke, 118–20
short-chain fatty acids (SCFAs), 109–11, 154, 181
Shrivastava, Amit, 156
Simon, Michele, 202
sleep, 157
smallpox, 15

smoking
emotional regulation and, 53
fetal development and, 55, 74, 80, 82, 90–91, 94–5, 172–3
NCDs and, 144
oxidative stress and, 151, 157–8
politics and, 196
poverty and, 172–3
type 2 diabetes and, 180
social anxiety disorder, 123
social brain, 45, 123, 130
social self, 133–5, 171
Southampton University, 84
Spalding, Kirsty, 88
specialised pro-resolving mediators (SPMs), 152, 160
sperm cells, 57, 63, 66
Sroufe, Alan, 39, 40
Start for Life, 210, 213
statins, 17
stem cells, 67–71
Stevens, Jane Ellen, 141
Still Face test, 130
Strandwitz, Philip, 132
Strange Situation test, 37
stress, 2, 105, 162–3, 215
chronic conditions and, 51–4
DNA methylation and, 26–7, 95
drug use and, 90–99, 128, 172
health habits and, 90–99, 128, 172–83
immune system and, 52–3, 111–12, 147–56
infancy and, 26, 44, 46–54, 123–35
inflammation and, 52–4, 151, 154, 163
microbiome and, 107, 175
oxytocin and, 123–7, 164–6
physical closeness and, 25, 123–35
poverty and, 167–91
pregnancy and, 48–9, 57, 74, 89–99
regulation and, 44–54, 125–35
relationships and, *see* relationships

275

Index

stress response
  diet and, 26, 174
  fetal alcohol syndrome and, 92
  poverty and, 171–2, 188, 208–9
  relationships and, 44, 49–52, 124, 127, 135, 147, 163–4
  response, 5, 46–52, 105
  separation from parents, 3, 49, 65, 128
  social self and, 134
strokes, 84, 98, 143, 144, 154, 160
sugar, 173–83
Suomi, Stephen, 128
Sure Start, 210, *211*, 213
Swami, Viren, 119
sympathetic nervous system, 47–8

T-cells, 109, 115–16, 164
television, 12
telomeres, 69
Theise, Neil, 70
Thompson, Amanda, 179
Thornburg, Kent, 98
timing, 40–43, 146
Tirado, Linda, 169, *169*, 170, 184
tongue tie, 117
tonsillitis, 115
training model, 36, 46, 212
transcription factors, 68
translational medicine approach, 29
type 1 diabetes, 109, 116, 146
type 2 diabetes, 3, 4, 17–18, 27, 29–30, 51, 57, 180–81, 183
  ACEs and, 154
  breastfeeding and, 116–17
  coronavirus and, 155–6
  fetal development and, 84–5, 98–9
  microbiome and, 154

United Nations, 197, 205
University of California, 89, 115
University of Colorado, 196
University of Minnesota, 164
University of Toulouse, 162
University of Turku, 161
upper lip tie, 117
Uvnas-Moberg, Kerstin, 165

vaccinations, 14–15, 115
vagal system, 5, 42, 44, 47n, 105, 129–33
Van de Vijver, Gertrudis, 25
van Tulleken, Chris, 122
Vareki, Saman, 205–6
vascular system, 76–7
Video Interaction Guidance (VIG), 212
Virginia Sterilization Act (1924), 20
vitamins, 76, 88, 151, 155
Volkow, Nora, 174

Wade, Nicholas, 22–3
Wadsworth, Michael, 55
Wahlbeck, Kristian, 190
Wallace, Alfred Russel, 55
Wang Xiaoyan, 116
Watch, Wait and Wonder, 212
Watson, James, 21
Webb, Beatrice and Sidney, 20
whole body systems, 70
whooping cough, 115
Williams, Robin, 171
Wolpert, Lewis, 68
World Economic Forum, 28
World Health Organization, 98

X-ray technology, 16

Zucchi, Fabiola, 50

About the Author

Sue Gerhardt is a British psychoanalytic psychotherapist. She has been awarded an honorary doctorate for her work in educating the public about neuroscience and child development. She was the co-founder, in 1998, of the Oxford Parent Infant Project, a charitable organisation that provides parent–infant psychotherapy to around fifty families each week. Sue's first book, the bestselling and critically acclaimed *Why Love Matters*, explained how affection shapes a child's brain in the first few months of life. Poignantly, she has also been diagnosed with Parkinson's disease, a condition thought to have some of its roots in infancy.